MALE
SEXUAL HEALTH

MALE
SEXUAL HEALTH

A Couple's Guide

Richard F. Spark, M.D.

Consumer Reports Books
A Division of Consumers Union
Yonkers, New York

Copyright © 1991 by Richard F. Spark
Published by Consumers Union of United States, Inc.,
Yonkers, New York 10703.

Library of Congress Cataloging-in-Publication Data
Spark, Richard F.
Male sexual health : a couple's guide / Richard F. Spark.
p.   cm.
Includes bibliographical references and index.
ISBN 0-89043-319-4 — ISBN 0-89043-318-6 (pbk.)
1. Impotence—Popular works.   I. Title.
RC889.S617   1991
616.6′92—dc20   90-26119
CIP

Design by GDS / Jeffrey L. Ward
Fourth printing, January 1993
Manufactured in the United States of America

Male Sexual Health is a Consumer Reports Book published by Consumers Union, the nonprofit organization that publishes *Consumer Reports*, the monthly magazine of test reports, product Ratings, and buying guidance. Established in 1936, Consumers Union is chartered under the Not-for-Profit Corporation Law of the State of New York.

The purposes of Consumers Union, as stated in its charter, are to provide consumers with information and counsel on consumer goods and services, to give information on all matters relating to the expenditure of the family income, and to initiate and to cooperate with individual and group efforts seeking to create and maintain decent living standards.

Consumers Union derives its income solely from the sale of *Consumer Reports* and other publications. In addition, expenses of occasional public service efforts may be met, in part, by nonrestrictive, noncommercial contributions, grants, and fees. Consumers Union accepts no advertising or product samples and is not beholden in any way to any commercial interest. Its Ratings and reports are solely for the use of the readers of its publications. Neither the Ratings nor the reports nor any Consumers Union publication, including this book, may be used in advertising or for any commercial purpose. Consumers Union will take all steps open to it to prevent such uses of its materials, its name, or the name of *Consumer Reports*.

To Barbara and our children,
Laura, Debra, Cynthia, and David

Contents

Acknowledgments

Many thanks to Dr. Thomas Stewart, chairman of the Department of Psychiatry at St. Raphael's Hospital in New Haven, Connecticut, for his thoughtful review and comments on Chapter 11, "Psychologic Factors Affecting Potency and Ejaculation."

Introduction:
The Problem

The scriptural directive is clear and unambiguous: "A man . . . shall cleave unto his wife and they shall be one flesh" (Genesis 1:23). For a man to cleave, his penis must swell and achieve an erection sufficient to allow for vaginal penetration. His penis remains firm during a period of thrusting until he ejaculates.

Men and women are unique in the animal kingdom. Most mammals are obliged to restrict their sexual activity to well-defined cycles when climate and availability of food and water are favorable for breeding. This is not true for the human species, for "that which distinguishes man from the beast is drinking without being thirsty and making love at all seasons" (*Le Mariage de Figaro*, Pierre de Beaumarchais). Some men cannot make love in any season because they are impotent. They can neither achieve nor sustain an erection satisfactory for intercourse. The loss of erectile function can have a profound effect on a man—and not only in the way he thinks about sex. The word *impotent* means lacking power or vigor, ineffective. Impotence can so undermine a man's self-esteem and confidence that it affects all his other relations with his partner, family members, and friends. Mistimed ejaculation or infertility can have similar consequences.

Approximately 20 to 30 million men in the United States suffer from impotence, either chronic or intermittent, yet an impotent man rarely discusses his problem—not even with his wife or sexual partner or his physician. Instead he becomes insular, reclusive, and defensive. This is understandable; until recently, medicine offered little reason for hope. A sense of failure and guilt, increasing self-doubt about one's masculinity, and depressive and even suicidal symptoms were natural consequences of the loss of potency.

Fortunately, this sense of doom is no longer warranted. In most cases, once the problem or problems responsible for impaired sexual function have been identified, physicians can develop effective treatments. What was once an arid therapeutic landscape is now awash with remedies.

Impotence is the most common sexual problem, but it is not the only one. Some men are potent but have premature or inhibited ejaculation. A growing number of men with normal potency and ejaculatory ability are infertile. *Male Sexual Health* explores these and other issues, describing and evaluating the full range of available treatments:

- For some impotent men, counseling to alleviate sexual anxieties suffices. Men with more complex emotional problems require more intensive individual psychotherapy.
- If the onset of sexual dysfunction coincided with the introduction of a new medication, substituting a different medicine may be all that is required for potency to return.
- When initial evaluation uncovers hormonal abnormalities, treatment directed at correcting the hormonal imbalance is most effective in restoring potency.
- Sexual dysfunction caused by an obstruction in genital blood flow can often be corrected with vascular surgery.
- Even a man with nerve damage can have erections by injecting a chemical into his penis.

• Still others may find that a penile prosthesis is best for their needs.

No single treatment is universally applicable to all impotent men. Whereas the proper therapeutic program results in restoration of male sexual and reproductive function with a gratifying success rate, other well-intentioned but inappropriate interventions are often ineffective, costly, and sometimes burdened with unacceptably high risks.

Male Sexual Health not only outlines the myriad problems responsible for disrupting male sexual and reproductive function but also describes, and then critically evaluates, the extensive array of new and traditional options now available to treat impotence and male infertility. Innovative techniques are now available to enhance sperm-ovum fusion, allowing many husbands to shed the designation "infertile male" for the more rewarding sobriquet "Daddy."

In a similar fashion new insights regarding the dynamics of sexual potency have expanded the scope of treatment for impotence. No single remedy is universally effective. It is still gratifying to note that entirely satisfactory results can be expected when treatment is targeted to correct a specific vascular, neurologic, hormonal, or psychologic problem. Optimal results often require a collaborative effort among the impotent man, his sexual partner, and the physician. Working together, they should be able to find within the realm of currently available therapeutic alternatives one that will allow them to enjoy a more satisfying sex life.

1

Changing Attitudes

Impotence is not a new problem; only our willingness to discuss it more openly is new. As far as we know, the topic was first described in detail in a biblical tale involving a king, a married woman, her husband, and a virgin.

David and Bathsheba, Uriah, and Abishag

David, slayer of Goliath, singer of psalms, and king of Judea, was a passionate man reputed to have ten concubines and several wives. Yet one day he grew restive and "arose from off his bed, and walked upon the roof of the king's house: and from the roof he saw a woman washing herself; and the woman was very beautiful to look upon." David was so stirred by the vision of Bathsheba that he summoned her to his chambers and "lay with her" and impregnated her.

Uriah, Bathsheba's husband and one of David's most loyal captains, was at the time waging war in a distant land. In an effort to disguise the paternity of Bathsheba's child, Uriah was summoned home. David assumed that Uriah would use the opportunity to sleep with Bathsheba. Then when her child was born, she could attribute the pregnancy to that union. But Uriah demurred. He would not even enter Bathsheba's house, let alone sleep with her, for like many men of his time, he believed that having intercourse sapped a man's strength, leaving him ill-prepared for battle.

When his ruse failed, David saw to it that Uriah was placed in a combat position that would inevitably result in his death. Only then could David take the widowed Bathsheba as his wife and claim to be the rightful father of his son, Solomon.

In the biblical account, David's action angered the Lord and he was punished. "Wherefore hast thou despised the commandment of the Lord, to do evil in his sight? Thou hast killed Uriah the Hittite with the sword, and has taken his wife to be thy wife" (II Samuel 12:9). David's sword was taken from him; he became despondent, ineffective, and impotent. In an effort to resurrect the king's flagging sexual function, David's advisers sent for a young virgin, Abishag, to rekindle his desires. "And the damsel was very fair, and cherished the king, and ministered to him: but the king knew her not" (I Kings 1:4). David had lost the power to have erections, and, by inference, it was presumed that he lacked the power to rule.

Why did David become impotent? The conventional biblical interpretation is that it was punishment for his philanderings with Bathsheba. Others argue that David, riddled with guilt over the entire affair and humiliated by his transgressions, became depressed, leading one to suspect that psychologic factors contributed to his sexual dysfunction (see chapter 11). It is also of some interest that David's impotence first occurred when he was seventy. Was it merely a natural consequence of aging? (See chapter 16.)

The story of David's impotence illustrates a prevalent attitude at that time: Man is naturally blessed with the gifts of potency and fertility and forfeits them only by his own indiscretions or the malicious acts of others.

Witches and Curses

The belief that impotence was caused by malicious acts became prominent during the Middle Ages, when the Church developed a proprietary interest in sexual dysfunction, primarily because impotence served as an impediment to procreation. The most thorough early descriptions of sexual problems and possible remedies appeared in the fifteenth century in *A Short Treatise About the People who, Impeded by Spells, are Unable to Have Intercourse with their Wives*. The text describes details of impotence-causing curses invoked by witches, including placement of "testicles of a cock under the bed." A sequence of remedies that might alleviate the spells includes ridding the house of diabolical substances, adequate confession, sprinkling the wall of the house with dog's blood, and carrying bile of fish. Finally, the text suggests that the couple abstain from intercourse for three days. Controlled abstinence is a recommendation still made today to alleviate a condition known as performance anxiety (see chapter 11).

Perhaps the most notorious medieval writing delving extensively into the problems of sexual function is the 1489 *Malleus Maleficarum*, or *The Witches Hammer*. The text is unequivocal: Impotence results from spells cast by witches under the direction of the devil. Here, too, a series of remedies are described, and if all fail, one may "approach the witch." Witch hunts followed.

By the sixteenth century, some people were beginning to consider that factors other than diabolical spells might be responsible for male sexual dysfunction. Dr. Johann Weyer, in 1563, speculated that impotence could result from natural causes or from the inappropriate use of medicines. This was the first indication that medication might impede sexual function (see chapter 9).

The Rooster Experiment

It was not until the nineteenth century that meaningful scientific inquiries into certain aspects of male sexual function were reported. In 1849 a German cleric, August Berthold, made critical observations by studying the behavior of common barnyard fowl. He noted that roosters chased hens but capons did not. (A capon is a rooster whose testicles have been removed to encourage development of tender flesh and a plump bird.) Berthold found that if he reimplanted testicles in the capon, the bird promptly resumed its innate roosterly behavior. This elegant and unusual avian experiment offered the first convincing evidence of a physiological role for the testicle in sexual function.

Forty years later the French neurologist Claude Brown-Sequard attempted to provide a clinical counterpart to Berthold's studies. He reported that he and other older men were revitalized by injections of watery extracts of animal testes. Since testosterone, the active hormonal component of the testis, is not water soluble, it remains unclear exactly what testicular products Dr. Brown-Sequard injected to achieve this salutary response. Perhaps the study served only to illustrate the confounding role of the placebo in the treatment of older men with diminished virility. Nevertheless, his experiments were the last scientific inquiries into the subject of male sexual function and dysfunction for decades. Other scientists working in this era found themselves oppressed by the stultifying influences of the Victorian Age, a period when investigation of matters relating to sex was neither encouraged nor condoned.

Freud and Oedipus

In the early twentieth century the overpowering influence of Sigmund Freud resurrected interest in sexual problems. Freud's achievements, although extraordinary, were so intimidating that they stifled research in other disciplines for a considerable period. Freud believed that men became impotent because they linked their sexual partners with their mothers, yet Freud himself had difficulty reconciling this concept with his own observations. He was convinced that all men experienced Oedipal conflict, but recognized that impotence was not universal.

Nonetheless, the belief that impotence was primarily a problem of *psychogenic* ("it's all in your head") origin dominated medical teaching until the early 1980s. Before that time it had been recognized that vascular, neurologic, and occasionally hormonal disorders might be associated with impaired sexual functioning. But prevailing dogma dictated that these physical disorders were rarely found in impotent men.

Today a more realistic appraisal stipulates that although psychologic factors unquestionably contribute to impotence in some instances, *physical* causes of impotence must also be considered. Psychological issues are critical, but they no longer supersede a comprehensive diagnostic evaluation to explore the possible role of such factors as nerve damage, problems with blood flow, hormone deficiencies, and side effects of medications.

The Whale and the Walrus

In the late 1930s and early 1940s, several physicians were preoccupied with the mechanics of the erectile process and tried to solve the problem of impotence by inserting a stiffening agent inside the flaccid penis of impotent males. Other mammals had solved this problem during evolution by developing a permanent bonelike structure within their erectile tissue. Referred to as an os-penis, this can acquire formidable dimensions. For example, the os-penis of the whale is six feet long, and a similar structure in the walrus is two feet in length.

Surgeons searching for a way to help men who had suffered penile mutilation decided to create a human os-penis. They were of the opinion that if one could endow the penis with permanent, rodlike firmness, then penetration of the vagina would always be possible. In 1936 two surgeons, one in Russia and the other in Germany, exploited this concept by using the cartilage from a man's rib to provide the penile rigidity required for vaginal penetration. Unfortunately, there were multiple technical problems with the cartilaginous implants, and the technique was soon abandoned. Still, this inventive surgical technique anticipated and heralded the future devel-

opment of the currently popular silicone penile prostheses
(see chapter 12).

It was the plight of individual men who had experienced
penile trauma that prompted surgical efforts to implant rib
cartilage. These physicians were unaware of the numbers of
nontraumatized healthy men who were unable to acquire
erections satisfactory for sexual intercourse. That information
emerged after the studies of Alfred Kinsey.

Kinsey

In 1948 Dr. Alfred Kinsey scandalized the public by publish-
ing *Sexual Behavior in the Human Male*. In this landmark
work Kinsey cataloged different patterns of male sexual function and reported that 2 percent of American men under the
age of forty suffered from impotence. His data implied that 10
million men were experiencing sexual problems. (These estimates were probably on the low side.) Despite his findings,
research into male sexual dysfunction proceeded slowly for
the next two decades.

The Turning Point

The early 1970s were watershed years. Researchers schooled
in disparate disciplines proved to be unusually productive and
broadened our basic knowledge of normal male sexual function. Each step forward led to the development of innovative
therapies for men suffering from impotence, ejaculatory disorders, or infertility.

Masters and Johnson

William Masters and Virginia Johnson studied the physiology
of sex by direct observation and, in 1970, published their
results, defining what they termed the normal male sexual
response cycle. Their innovative treatment for sexual dysfunction involved both partners in several weeks of specific

exercises to restore sexual communication, intimacy, and satisfaction (see chapter 11).

The Vascular Steal Syndrome

Medical research had been making strides in related areas. A French surgeon, Dr. R. Leriche, discovered that when severe atherosclerosis (hardening of the arteries) partially blocked some branches of the abdominal aorta, the normal flow of blood into the penis did not occur. In 1973 Czechoslovakian surgeon Dr. V. Michal described a somewhat different vascular problem, which he termed the pelvic steal syndrome. In this disorder, a man can acquire and sustain an erection as long as he doesn't move his legs. Moving the legs drains—"steals"—blood away from the pelvis, so the erection collapses. This type of impotence can now be corrected with surgery that unblocks the affected artery. Then blood can flow freely to the genitalia and remain there throughout intercourse. Other forms of impotence due to blood vessel blockage are now attributed to impaired blood flow through still smaller blood vessels. This, too, can be corrected by surgery (see chapter 7).

Erections and the Electroencephalogram

Neurologists, aware of the role of the central, peripheral, and autonomic nervous systems in erectile process, provided new insights into the neurophysiology of erections. It had long been known that most men wake in the morning with an erection. Although the erection occurs coincident with a full bladder, and disappears after urination, filling the bladder with urine does not cause the erection. Rather, this early-morning erection is associated with specific electrical changes occurring in the brain during sleep.

Most men, independent of sexual desire, experience spontaneous erections while sleeping. These nocturnal erections coincide with the onset of a particular type of sleep called rapid-eye-movement (REM) sleep. Using an electroenceph-alogram (EEG), which measures electrical activity in the brain, and direct observation, physicians can monitor the brain-wave patterns identifying the onset of REM sleep and the appearance of erections. The procedure, referred to as nocturnal penile tumescence (NPT) monitoring, is one diag-nostic test often employed in the early evaluation of men complaining of impotence. Other neural reflexes critical to erection can also be assessed by direct testing to determine whether there is an underlying neurological cause for im-paired erectile function (see chapter 6).

Urologists "Cut to the Chase"

Another critical development in the early 1970s involved two groups of urologic surgeons who independently proposed that the most direct way to help men suffering from impotence was to unburden them of the anxiety associated with first acquiring and then sustaining an erection satisfactory for intercourse. The urologists reasoned that if they provided the man's flaccid penis with a mechanical device that gives it permanent rodlike firmness, vaginal penetration could be achieved on demand, independent of sexual desire or arousal. In essence, this de-vice would allow men to be perpetually prepared for sexual intercourse. At the same time, silicone became readily avail-able, and the first penile prostheses were developed and im-planted (see chapter 12).

The Pulsating Hypothalamus

In the same decade, two pivotal developments in the field of endocrinology once again emphasized the role of hormones in normal male sexual function. Researchers identified and ana-lyzed a new hormone, gonadotropin releasing hormone (GnRH). GnRH is made in a portion of the brain called the hypothalamus, from which the hormonal regulation of male sexual function is orchestrated. Later, it was determined that the pattern of GnRH release is critical; "pulsatile GnRH secretion" is a prerequisite for male sexual and reproductive success.

Further Advances in Endocrinology

By the early 1980s my colleagues and I had accumulated enough experience to publish "Impotence Is Not Always Psychogenic." In a group of 105 men with complaints of impotence, we found thirty-five who had specific hormonal abnormalities. Recognition of the abnormality and institution of appropriate treatment resulted in prompt restoration of potency. By the end of the decade, the role of the pituitary gland and of a portion of the brain called the temporal lobe as regulators of male sexual function was appreciated (see chapter 8).

Help Is Available

Physicians in many specialties are now equipped to take initial exploratory steps in diagnosing male sexual problems. Then, if necessary, an extensive network of subspecialists is available to help. Detailed evaluation and effective treatment can be developed in collaboration with doctors trained in urology, sexual therapy, or endocrinology.

2

You Are Not Alone

When a man is unable to achieve an erection satisfactory for intercourse, he is considered impotent. Many men, if not all men, have at one time or another experienced isolated episodes of impotence. Often this is transient, a result of fatigue, excessive drinking, or preoccupation with business or family problems. Under these circumstances it would be inappropriate to saddle the man with a diagnosis of complete impotence; instead he is said to have experienced situational erectile dysfunction. Criteria established by Masters and Johnson indicate that a diagnosis of impotence is appropriate only when a man experiences failure more than 25 percent of the time during attempted intercourse.

How Common Is Impotence?

It was not until the middle of the twentieth century that reliable information on the prevalence of impotence was available. As previously noted, Dr. Alfred Kinsey, in his *Sexual Behavior in the Human Male*, estimated that impotence occurred in less than 2 percent of men under the age of forty. The incidence increased gradually with age, so that, according to Kinsey, 6.7 percent of men were impotent by age fifty-five and almost 25 percent at seventy. Recent data suggest that Kinsey's report significantly underestimated the total. Current surveys indicate that impotence plagues 20 to 30 million American men.

Part of the problem in collecting accurate data relates to men's lack of candor when discussing sexual problems. Most men are more than willing to answer questions about their income, general health, and smoking and drinking habits. They are often disarmingly frank about their extramarital relationships, sexual preferences, and sex life. Still, the same men are recalcitrant when confronted with a questionnaire asking for truthful and accurate answers regarding sexual impairment. In these times of extraordinary sexual enlightenment, impotence may be the only subject remaining in the closet.

Because it is important to have some estimate of the prevalence of impotence, investigators have devised a series of questionnaires with sufficient ingenuity to provide information that may have been overlooked in the past.

For example, two investigators, Drs. Anthony Reading and William Weist, recruited subjects in London, England, by proposing to examine attitudes relating to the development of a male contraceptive. During the course of the extensive interview, information was elicited relative to the volunteers' current sexual function and dysfunction. The investigators found that among a group of presumably healthy, sexually active, heterosexual Englishmen (age twenty to thirty-five) involved in a stable relationship, 8.25 percent admitted having difficulty achieving and maintaining an erection satisfactory for sexual intercourse and 18.5 percent said that they did not achieve an erection satisfactory for masturbation.

Dr. Ellen Frank and her associates at the University of Southern California decided that the optimal way to verify descriptions of male sexual function was to direct the same questions to *both* husband and wife. Dr. Frank, like others, recognized that reliable descriptions of sexual function are most likely to be obtained from a subtle approach. Her extensive fifteen-page questionnaire, therefore, contained only one and one-half pages relating to sex. In her survey of one hundred married couples in their mid-thirties, Dr. Frank identified surprisingly high levels of sexual dysfunction reported by the men and confirmed by their wives. Sixteen percent of the men reported difficulty acquiring or sustaining an erection. In addition, 36 percent felt they ejaculated too quickly, and 4 percent were unable to ejaculate at all. This number is roughly twenty times Kinsey's estimate for a similar age group.

Dr. Michael Slag of the Minneapolis Veterans Administration expanded on Frank's observations, providing data from a different perspective. He interviewed men attending a Veterans Administration outpatient clinic for problems unrelated to sexual function and found that of 1,180 men, 401 (34 percent) complained of impotence. But this patient population differed in several respects from the couples studied by Dr. Frank.

The men in Dr. Slag's study were older; the average age was fifty. In addition, all had some medical problem that prompted them to visit the clinic. In many cases the illness itself was the primary cause of sexual dysfunction. It is also worth noting that men attending any clinic can be expected to receive medication, and many medications can affect sexual function. In fact, Dr. Slag was able to incriminate medications as a direct cause of the impotence in 22 percent of the impotent men in this study.

Dr. Leslie Schover, a psychologist at the State University of New York at Stony Brook, surveyed 300 men with a mean age of 55 and reported that 21 percent of them complained of impotence.

On the basis of all studies available to date, it now appears that approximately 10 percent of healthy men under the age of forty and probably 20 to 35 percent of those under the age of sixty experience some form of sexual dysfunction.

Does Aging Contribute to Impotence?

Kinsey's observation that older men experience problems with sex more often than younger men is accurate. But the reasons remain the subject of considerable controversy. Gerontologists have been studying a group of healthy older men age sixty to seventy-nine as part of the Baltimore Longitudinal Study (BLS) on aging. Men in the study were queried about their sexual activity during the course of a year. They were then divided into those who had "least," "medium," and "most" sexual events (intercourse and/or masturbation). Roughly equal numbers of men fell into each category. This suggested that some independent factor—not age alone—determines the level of sexual vigor for men over sixty. In this population of healthy men, only 25 to 35 percent reported difficulty achieving a functional erection.

Other investigators have challenged the BLS observations, maintaining that they are not reproducible. Dr. Alexander Vermeulen of Belgium arrived at a diametrically opposed conclusion. His data indicate that among sixty- to eighty-year-old men, only 25 to 35 percent do *not* have problems; fully 65 to 75 percent do. Some argue that it is not the aging process per se but other concomitant factors that are responsible for the diminished sexual ability of older men. The BLS study may be faulted because only men who were unusually healthy and free of common medical problems such as high blood pressure and diabetes mellitus qualified for inclusion. Since both high blood pressure and diabetes are common in older men, many investigators believe it is inappropriate to generalize observations from the BLS experience to other geriatric populations.

Effects of Hypertension, Diabetes, and Medications

High blood pressure (hypertension) by itself has a negative effect on male sexual activity. Untreated hypertensive men are three times more likely to experience potency problems than men of similar age with normal blood pressure. Unfortunately, antihypertensive medication can cause further deterioration in erectile or ejaculatory function.

To overcome problems caused by medications, the patient can describe the unpleasant and unwanted effects to his physician in detail (being forthright about potency problems) and the physician can adjust drug dosage or prescribe alternative medication to control high blood pressure without negative sexual (and other) side effects. The same approach holds true for many other medications routinely used to treat a spectrum of common problems such as peptic ulcer, gastrointestinal disturbances, depression, and a wide range of psychiatric conditions. Many of these can interfere with normal erections (see Chapter 9, "Medications, Chemicals, and Potency," for a comprehensive list of prescription medications and chemicals that adversely affect male sexual function).

Diabetes mellitus can have a devastating effect on a man's sexual function. As many as 35 percent of diabetic men twenty to sixty years old experience impotence, whereas only 9 to 10 percent of nondiabetic age-matched controls are similarly affected.

Diabetes is associated with an increased predisposition to two types of vascular disease. One affects the large blood vessels that supply blood to the pelvis. The other involves the smaller blood vessels in the penis that must dilate to become engorged with blood so that an erection can occur. If an impotent, diabetic man has evidence of either macro- or microvascular disease in body organs distant from the genital area (heart, eyes, kidney, etc.), he most likely has vasculogenic impotence.

Diabetic patients are also prone to nerve damage (neuropathy) throughout the nervous system. When this occurs, these men lose the critical processes involved in stimulating erections and are considered to have neurogenic impotence.

Effective treatment depends on pinpointing the specific defect responsible for the erectile failure; treatment for vasculogenic impotence differs from that for neurogenic impotence.

Prevention of Impotence

There is no way to stave off aging, but some modifications in behavior can help minimize risks of sexual dysfunction. Smoking, heavy drinking, obesity, high levels of serum cholesterol, and elevated blood sugar levels, as well as the use of narcotic or other mood-altering drugs, can all contribute to impotence. Early investments in weight reduction, temperance in alcohol consumption, and avoidance of nicotine and drugs during youth may provide significant sexual dividends later on.

3

What Is Normal?

It is tempting to think of sexual intercourse as a seamless process flowing effortlessly from arousal to erection to ejaculation. This level of understanding suffices only for those men fortunate enough never to have experienced sexual problems. The events included in the normal male sexual response cycle are complex and depend on orchestrated events that involve the brain and the nervous, vascular, and hormonal systems.

The cycle of male sexual response may be partitioned into six components: libido, erection, plateau, ejaculation and orgasm, detumescence, and refractory period. The proper sequencing and integration of these phases is critical.

- *Libido* describes the intensity of sexual desire or drive.
- *Erection* refers to the transition of the penis from a limp to an erect state. Increased blood flow into specialized chambers in the penis is necessary for this transition to occur. Nerve signals that originate in the spinal cord are responsible for activating increased blood flow.

- The *plateau* phase occurs at the peak of sexual excitement and is associated with increases in pulse, blood pressure, and respiration rate.
- *Ejaculation*, the pulsatile release of semen, is entirely under neurologic control. *Orgasm* is the pleasurable feeling and sense of relaxation following ejaculation.
- *Detumescence* is the loss of erection after ejaculation.
- During the *refractory period* men are unable to acquire another erection.

Libido

Psychologic factors and the hormone testosterone, which is produced by the testicles, regulate male libido. Studies in animals have demonstrated that removal of the testicles results in a precipitous decline in testosterone levels in the bloodstream. Shortly thereafter, the castrated animal loses sexual interest.

Some impotent men have testicles that cannot produce adequate amounts of testosterone; they have lower than normal serum testosterone levels. These men notice a gradual but progressive diminution in sexual desire. Potency may be preserved during brief interludes of subnormal serum testosterone levels, but when testosterone production remains chronically low, impotence is inevitable. Treatment with testosterone usually restores sexual desire and potency.

Emotional setbacks as a result of clinical depression, loss of a loved one, or a business reversal can also result in a decline in libido. For these men, whose testosterone levels are normal, testosterone treatment is neither warranted nor effective. Rather, recognition and treatment of the depression, the grief, or the self-doubts are more appropriate. Counseling or psychotherapy is often helpful in restoring sexual desire.

Erection

Men acquire erections by fantasy or when confronted with erotic stimuli (psychogenic erections), after direct stimulation of their genitals (reflex erections), and spontaneously during sleep (nocturnal erections).

Psychogenic erections occur in response to any one of a variety of sensory stimuli, usually visual or auditory. Visual and auditory cues are so reliably consistent in provoking psychogenic erections that behavioral therapists often use them to learn more about what stimulates or inhibits erections in normal and sexually dysfunctional men.

All such studies share a traditional experimental "stimulus-response" design. The stimulus is either an audio- or videotape describing or showing heterosexual sex acts. The response is an erection, which is recorded by attaching a sensor, somewhat like a blood pressure cuff, to the volunteer's penis. The device measures changes in penis size and can be used to determine what conditions enhance or inhibit erection. A normally potent man exposed to an erotic audio- or videotape will develop an erection. When, for example, the content of the audiotape is held constant but the subject is distracted and asked to complete an innocuous questionnaire, he loses his erection. Similarly, if the videotape is replaced by a neutral travelogue, the subject loses his erection.

This stimulus-response model has provided some predictable as well as some unexpected insights into the interaction between psychological influences and physical responses. The observation that for heterosexual men an audiotape narrated by a female is more effective in provoking an erection than a similar script narrated by a male is not surprising. Less intuitive is the observation that although mildly threatening cues result in diminution of the erection, increasing the intensity of the threatening stimulus enhances arousal.

Neural Connections

Two centers in the spinal cord serve as important junctions for psychogenic and reflex erections (see figure 1). The first site, located in the upper back, is the thoracolumbar erection center. It appears to be a critical way station for psychogenic

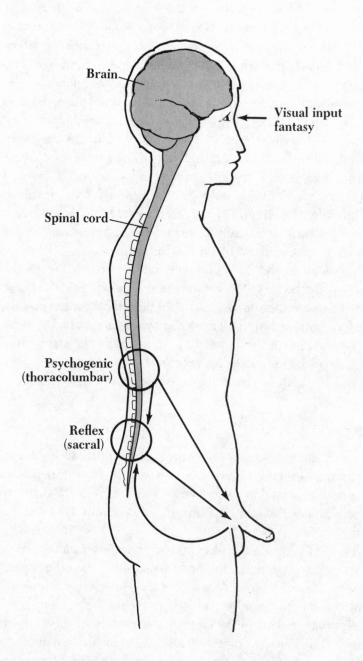

Figure 1. Sites of spinal cord erection centers for psychogenic (thoracolumbar) and reflex (sacral) erections.

erections. The second site, in the lower back, or sacrum, is the sacral erection center. Nerve routes from this area receive and send impulses to the genitalia to facilitate reflex erections.

Reflex erections are initiated by local nerve impulses originating in the genital area. Manual or oral stimulation of the penis or scrotum will evoke a reaction in bundles of nerve fibers in the penis called pacinian corpuscles, activating the first segment of a reflex circuit. (The tip, or glans, of the penis contains the greatest concentration of these pressure-sensitive corpuscles.) Neural impulses arising in local or genital nerves travel with lightning speed to the lower spine. Once received at this site, the circuit is completed by transmission of nerve messages back to the genital nerves to set in motion a series of events that increase blood flow into the penis.

Still another set of neurologic signals originating in the lower spine travel to the prostate and seminal vesicles. These structures are the source of seminal fluid that is released during ejaculation. Impulses from the lower sacral areas also activate muscles in the pelvis to help maintain the strength of both psychogenic and reflex erections. The same muscles will be called on later to contract rhythmically during ejaculation.

Vascular Reactions

The foregoing describes the neurologic connections necessary for normal erectile function. The actual process depends on events that stimulate blood vessels in the penis to dilate to accommodate the massive influx of blood required for an erection.

The penis contains three cylindrical bundles of blood vessels (two corpora cavernosa and one corpus spongiosum) uniquely designed to trap blood (see figure 2). The spongy tissues fill and become engorged with blood to create the erection.

Normally, when blood flows into a portion of the body, it enters and exits promptly, providing nourishment and removing wastes. This inflow and outflow is efficient for all or-

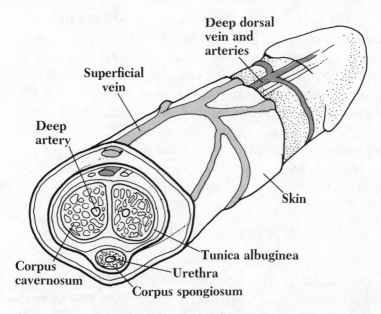

Figure 2. Cross section of penis showing location of erectile cylinders (corpus cavernosum and corpus spongiosum).

gans of the body but is not conducive to the development and maintenance of an erection. Blood must flow into, and be held captive within, the penile corporal bodies to allow for initial swelling. Then another process must inhibit outflow so that a rigid erection develops and is maintained: Small blood vessels in the penis swell and exert pressure on the veins that normally allow blood to drain out of the penis. The blood in the penis is "trapped," and the erection can be maintained until orgasm or stimulation ceases.

Plateau

Following erection, most men reach a plateau. During the plateau phase, which may last from thirty seconds to two minutes, a rapid series of events occurs.

Men experience a flushing of the face and an increase in

heart rate up to 150 to 175 beats per minute. At the same time, distinct rises in both systolic (pressure when heart contracts) and diastolic (pressure in between heart contractions) blood pressure are evident. Testicular size increases by 50 percent. Then, fluid from the accessory sexual organs, the prostate and seminal vesicles, begins to discharge. This preclimactic stage is under neural control and prepares the man for ejaculation. Signals from the nervous system facilitate the movement of sperm-rich fluid from the seminal vesicles and prostate into the urethra in anticipation of ejaculation.

Ejaculation and Orgasm

Ejaculation and orgasm occur as pelvic muscles contract to propel seminal fluid through and out the urethra. The urethra is a hollow tube in the center of the penis that allows urine to be eliminated from the bladder. At the culmination of sexual excitement, carefully timed neurologic impulses act to close the internal bladder valve (sphincter). This allows all the ejaculated seminal fluid to be pushed *forward* through the urethra (antegrade ejaculation).

If the bladder sphincter does not close, ejaculated semen is forced *backward* into the bladder. This abnormal ejaculation, called retrograde ejaculation, occurs in some paraplegics, in men treated with some antihypertensive medications (such as guanethidine), and often after prostate or bladder surgery or radiation treatment to the pelvis. Men who lose the capacity to have antegrade ejaculation can retain erectile function and experience orgasm, but they often become alarmed when they do not sense fluid passing through the urethra. Some become depressed over their inability to complete this phase of the male sexual response cycle. Impotence may follow.

Orgasm is distinct from ejaculation. Orgasm is the pleasurable phenomenon experienced at a conscious level that is associated with the rhythmic contraction of certain pelvic muscles (the bulbocavernosus and ischiocavernosus muscles); a sense of relaxation follows.

Detumescence and Refractory Period

Following ejaculation, blood drains out of the penis, which then reverts to its normal resting state. The penis remains flaccid for a period of time during which neither erection nor ejaculation is possible. The penis is considered to be unresponsive (refractory) to stimulation during this interval. The duration of the refractory period seems to vary with age; younger men may experience reflexogenic erections thirty to forty-five minutes after ejaculation, whereas older men may require two to three hours or more.

4

Defining the Problem

Men who become impotent tend to concentrate their energy and anxiety on a recalcitrant penis that does not become erect when it should. But riveting attention on the penis is not the best way to resolve the problem.

What is perceived solely as an inability to achieve an erection may in fact be traced to a specific problem in one of three phases (libido, erection, ejaculation) of the normal male sexual response cycle. Psychiatrists, psychologists, and sex therapists use a language that differs slightly from the terminology used in this book. In their vernacular, *sexual desire* takes the place of libido; *arousal* is used instead of erection; and *orgasm* is substituted for ejaculation.

There are several avenues through which these individual areas of sexual vulnerability can be explored. Only by teasing apart the individual components of the male sexual response cycle can the cause of ongoing sexual failure be revealed. Then a focused treatment plan can be formulated.

Desire Phase (Libido) Problems

Two desire phase problems, low sexual desire or aversion to sex, are now recognized. When psychologists and sex therapists talk about low sexual desire, they do so in a global fashion. If a man complains of reduced desire, it is important to know whether it is partner specific. Has the man lost interest in having sex only with his partner? Does he have any interest in, or fantasize about, having sex with other partners? Is he having erotic dreams? Does he have any sexual fantasies? Do spontaneous erections occur under any circumstances?

If the answer is yes to any of the above, the diagnosis is not low sexual desire. That diagnosis is reserved for men who answer no to all these questions. Men with genuine low sexual desire often state that they cannot remember the last time they experienced any sensation of lust, horniness, or true sexual desire.

Low Sexual Desire

Four readily recognizable events—death of a spouse, physical illness, recent surgery, and divorce—result in a predictable loss of sexual desire. Blunting of desire is also a common but transient phenomenon after any physically or emotionally stressful episode. The sexual problems of men who have suffered an acute medical illness or recent surgery are, for the most part, of limited duration. Desire and potency will return slowly but steadily. For widowers and divorced men, the sequence of events is more protracted but usually resolves with time alone or limited reassurance and counseling.

In other instances, the precipitating factors responsible for the loss of sexual desire are less apparent. Additional effort is required to unravel the chain of events that singly or collectively served to quench the libido.

A lack or progressive diminution in sexual desire may also be the harbinger of depression. Depressions are complex medical problems and require more detailed evaluation and treatment. Potency returns to depressed men only when their depression is alleviated. Often antidepressant medications are necessary to help cope with symptoms of depression (see chapter 11).

Aversion to Sex

Aversion to sex is an uncommon and poorly understood subcategory of impaired sexual desire. This diagnosis implies not just a lack of interest in sex but an overall repugnance about all sexual activities. The man suffering from sexual aversion finds sex a disgusting, anxiety-provoking experience and the cause of severe guilt and shame. Aversion to sex is often reported by men with primary impotence (men who have never been potent). It is rarely seen in the man with secondary impotence (a man who was potent in the past but is now having difficulty achieving erections), though it may occur if he discovers a shift in gender preference. Recently recognized homosexual feelings may evoke a so-called selective impotence, and he develops an aversion to sex with females only.

Arousal Phase Disorders

Psychologists classify problems achieving and sustaining erections as arousal phase disorders. Men with inadequate arousal insist that they have normal desire, a persistent passionate sexual feeling. They complain primarily of the inability either to achieve or to maintain an erection satisfactory for sexual intercourse. They are frequently troubled by the fact that they don't enjoy sex as much as they used to.

It is important to determine whether the impotent man still has erections and, if so, under what circumstances. Normally, erections occur spontaneously during sleep. He may be aware of his spontaneous nighttime erections only when he wakes up in the morning and finds that his penis is fully erect. This implies that the neurologic signals and blood flow to the penis are still operating normally. REM sleep seems to be critical for the initiation of early morning erections. Men who sleep fitfully will not have erections when they wake in the morning; this is no cause for alarm.

If a well-rested man does not have erections when he arises, it is important to determine whether he can get an erection under any other circumstances. Can he bring his penis to an erection when masturbating? Does his penis become erect when he views sexually explicit material or an erotic film? Is there someone other than his wife who can stimulate him to an erection? If the answer is yes to any of those questions, blood flow (vascular) and neurologic signals to the genitals are likely intact.

The ability to have a brief, but not lasting, erection is characteristic of men who have penile venous incompetence. With this condition, the blood vessels fail to close off the veins that carry blood from penile chambers, so that the blood drains from the penis shortly after the initial erection is achieved. The problem can be corrected by surgery. However, surgery is not necessary for all men who have difficulty maintaining an erection.

Sometimes erections occur and then disappear as the man loses concentration on the sexual act. This so-called lack of sensate focus is common in middle-age men. It can be corrected relatively easily with a series of sensate focus exercises described in Chapter 11, "Psychologic Factors Affecting Potency and Ejaculation."

Many older men have difficulty acquiring an erection and become disheartened when it seems to fade prior to penetration. Surgery is not necessary for these men either. Continued local genital stimulation generally restores erectile vigor.

An unusual medical condition referred to as Peyronie's disease may eventually cause the erect penis to bend into a J shape that renders it virtually useless for intercourse. The growth of fibrous bands in the outer sheaf (or tunica albuginea) of the penis is responsible for the deviation in shape. This can be repaired by surgery to release restricting bands or, as a last resort, by insertion of a penile prosthesis.

Men who are unable to have an erection with a partner often have spontaneous erections during sleep or in the early morning. This is vital information because it indicates that both neurologic reflexes and blood flow to the penis are adequate. The selective erectile failure may be a manifestation of performance anxiety, a common condition usually amenable to treatment through counseling or sensate focus exercises (see chapter 11).

Orgasm Phase Problems

Orgasm phase axis problems include premature, inhibited, or retrograde ejaculation.

Premature Ejaculation

It is often difficult to determine exactly when ejaculation is premature, for in nature the ability to ejaculate rapidly is valued, and in the animal world rapid ejaculation after vaginal penetration is a desirable trait. Such activity ensures an efficient evolution of the species and also allows the coupling creatures to spend little time in the defenseless posture of sexual intercourse. As soon as their reproductive act is completed, they can go on with the more critical business of day-to-day living, like foraging for food and defending against predators.

Such is not the case with man, for the advent of the supermarket has greatly simplified food gathering, and if one discounts the distracting influence of a small child at the bedroom door requesting a glass of water, no meaningful predators threaten extended human sexual activity.

Certainly ejaculation can be considered premature if it occurs prior to vaginal penetration. Thereafter, the precise amount of thrusting time necessary to achieve ejaculation varies. From a *reproductive* perspective, no problem exists as long as ejaculation occurs intravaginally. In terms of the sensual experience, couples find that a more prolonged period of intravaginal pelvic thrusting prior to ejaculation maximizes sexual excitement and increases opportunities for female orgasm. Exercises can condition men to put off ejaculation for a longer period. Such "squeeze" and "start-stop" techniques are discussed in detail on page 136.

Inhibited Ejaculation

Some men who are able to have erections cannot ejaculate. The condition responsible for this may be readily apparent. Paraplegic men cannot ejaculate because the nerves in the spinal cord responsible for ejaculation have been destroyed. A common side effect of many antidepressant medications is an inability to ejaculate. The ejaculatory nerves remain intact, but they are inactivated.

Spinal cord injuries and antidepressants are not the only causes of an inability to ejaculate. Psychologic factors can play a prominent role. Delayed or inhibited ejaculation is often attributed to a man's subconscious desire to withhold something valuable from his sexual partner. The reasons for this vary, but usually involve a man's repressed anger toward his sexual partner. Withholding semen by inhibiting ejaculation is one means of establishing absolute and ultimate control during the sexual act.

Problems arise when a man perceives, rightly or wrongly, that he alone has been forced to shoulder what should have been a mutual burden. A partner's lack of support or interest in the midst of a career crisis, a failure to share the anguish of a serious illness in a family member, or the inability to recognize a man's need to be engaged in some meaningful work even when retired are among the areas of conflict identified in men who are unable to ejaculate.

Therapy directed at understanding and rooting out the underlying disaffection toward the sexual partner is usually effective in allowing the normal ejaculatory process to resume.

Retrograde Ejaculation

A woman may believe that her partner has not ejaculated if she does not sense a pulse of semen in her vagina at the conclusion of intercourse. What she perceives as a lack of ejaculation may in fact be only a loss of the ability to ejaculate forward. Some men experience orgasm and ejaculate, but the semen they ejaculate squirts *backward* into their bladder (retrograde ejaculation) instead of *forward* through their penis (antegrade ejaculation). This is a common occurrence in men who have had prostate or bladder surgery or radiation treatments to the pelvis.

Retrograde ejaculation is also a problem for hypertensive men who are treated with the antihypertensive medication guanethidine (Ismelin). In contrast, some medications useful in the treatment of depression and low sexual desire may restore sexual desire and the ability to achieve erections. But they do so at the expense of the ability to ejaculate (see chapter 10).

5

Finding the Cause

When a man's sexual function declines, all he knows is that he can't perform and he wants treatment to get the problem fixed right away. Treatment follows diagnosis. The medical history, a series of directed questions, is the first step in the diagnostic process. To find out whether a man's sexual dysfunction is physical or psychologic in nature, the physician starts by exploring the circumstances surrounding a man's transition from a potent to an impotent state. Details of his current and past erectile and ejaculatory function are reviewed, along with general health issues. The medical history format may vary among physicians, but the questions and their rationales remain remarkably constant. Men experiencing sexual problems can expect to discuss these issues with their doctors and should anticipate how they will respond.

The Medical History

When did your sexual problems begin?

For most men, sexual problems evolve as an insidious stuttering process characterized by intermittent loss and restoration of sexual function over several years. As the condition responsible for the original sexual failure becomes more firmly entrenched, a man struggles to maintain some sexual interest and potency. Eventually he experiences a complete loss of sexual capabilities.

At times an impotent man may describe a different scenario and give a history of sudden loss of sexual potency that then becomes persistent and unremitting.

"I can tell you the exact date and time that the problem happened. It was 11:00 P.M. on my wife's birthday. Four months earlier, on my birthday, sexual function was fine. When her birthday rolled around, I was unable to perform and have been unable to get an erection from that date on."

Psychologic problems are the most likely cause of impotence for this man and other men with similar histories. With the exception of acute penile or spinal cord trauma, no physical or physiologic process causes a sudden and permanent disappearance of male sexual function.

When was the last time your sexual function was normal?

Men with sexual problems are frequently so despondent about their loss of potency that they cannot recall a moment when their sexual function was normal. The definition of "normal" also may be elusive. A man of sixty may feel that sexual function was truly satisfactory only when he was in his twenties and capable of prodigious feats of sexual prowess. If he expects treatment to allow him to recapture the sexual glory of his youth, he will be disappointed. A more reasonable baseline estimate for normal sexual function can be obtained by reviewing his level of sexual activity five to seven years ago. It is possible that during those years he considered sexual function satisfactory if he could make love about once a week or even once every two weeks. If he has no sexual capability now, a more appropriate therapeutic goal may be to aim for a return to weekly or biweekly sexual intercourse.

Do you still have erections?

If a man has fully rigid erections during sleep, when he wakes up in the morning, or under any circumstances, the doctor will assume that the neurologic impulses for triggering an erection and the vascular channels leading to the penile erectile cylinders are intact. If, on the other hand, erections are totally absent, then nerve damage or vascular insufficiency must be suspected. Erections that occur briefly and then fade suggest other diagnoses, including penile venous incompetence (see chapter 7), lack of sensate focus (see chapter 11), or presbyrectia (see chapter 16). Treatments are available for all of these conditions.

Have your feelings toward your partner changed?

Conflict sets the stage for a common, usually reversible, type of male sexual dysfunction. Squabbles, disagreements, and arguments are an inevitable component of any close relationship. Discussion, mediation, some old-fashioned bellowing, or even weeping may be called into play to arrive at a satisfactory resolution. Not all discord is resolved to each partner's satisfaction.

When waters churned up during an argument are eventually stilled, the calm may be confined to the surface. Bruised feelings, submerged in the interest of restoring harmony, do not disappear; they linger to fester in the fertile fields of the subconscious. It is here, in the subconscious, that gnawing anger, insecurities, and resentments form a powerful coalition to cripple male sexual function.

Sometimes the areas of conflict seem almost childish and superficial.

Sam was fifty-two years old and had been impotent for about three years. The circumstances surrounding the development of his impotence were not apparent to him at first, but after reflecting about it he recalled that just before the age of fifty

he had a passionate desire to own a sports car at a cost some-
where in excess of $40,000. He discussed this with his wife,
who pointed out that they could not afford that sort of indul-
gence. Not swayed by her logic, he countered that he had
worked hard all his life, sacrificed for others, and now, as he
was approaching fifty, was entitled to this one little luxury.
Apparently her rejoinder was something like, "A little luxury?
A car like that is nothing but a penis extender for small boys."
From that moment on he was unable to have an erection.

Is there someone else?

Not all relationships are forever. When a married man finds
himself attracted to another woman and engages in an extramarital affair, he may remain fully potent with his wife and
mistress, or he may reserve his potency for his mistress and
display a selective impotence with his wife. Only when he has
sexual problems with both his wife and mistress will he feel
compelled to seek medical assistance. Guilt is usually responsible for his impotence. The dynamics are not complex.

A man may be attracted to the other woman because she is
younger, slimmer, prettier, sexier, or just different from his
wife. He is consumed with but also ashamed of his passion for
her. Potency can be restored only by resolving his guilt. Counseling or therapy can be helpful for this and other forms of
impotence caused by emotional or psychologic conflict. Treatment, however, is effective only if the man is willing to accept
the notion that the therapeutic process is, first, not a threat
to his masculinity and, second, will take some time, usually
several months, before positive results can be achieved.

Have you been under unusual stress?

A variety of life stresses associated with work, job insecurity,
financial pressure, personal strife, or an illness in a family
member can consume so much of a man's attention that he
becomes preoccupied with his worries and loses all interest in

intimate sexual activity. Onerous daily burdens drain sexual energy and must be disposed of so that he can recapture and refocus his sexual life. This plan is more readily outlined than implemented.

Do you have any problem with ejaculation?

Discharge of semen out of the penis sooner than expected or desired is referred to as premature ejaculation. Ordinarily, ejaculation occurs only after a prolonged period of intravaginal penile thrusting. Ideally the duration of thrusting will be sufficient to allow the man and his partner to achieve orgasm at about the same time. Ejaculation that occurs immediately after penetration minimizes both male and female sexual pleasure.

Exercises are available to allow the man to contain his ejaculate for a longer period of time. The so-called squeeze and start-stop techniques are discussed in chapter 11.

An inability to ejaculate is another source of concern. Some medications routinely used in the treatment of the common cold, nasal congestion, and depression inhibit the reflexes that allow ejaculation to occur. Cold medications can be abandoned, but antidepressant drugs are not so readily discarded. Adjustment in the type of antidepressant drug prescribed may help restore normal ejaculation.

Is ejaculation painful?

Some men experience pain when they ejaculate. The anticipation of intense pain with ejaculation is understandably a powerful disincentive to sex. Ejaculatory pain originates in the rectum and passes like a bolt of electricity through the penis at the moment of orgasm. An inflammation or infection in the prostate is often responsible. Treatment with antibiotics or warm baths usually diminishes the inflammation and infection and allows ejaculation to occur without pain.

Is there blood in your semen?

The sudden appearance of bloody seminal fluid is an alarming symptom requiring prompt medical attention and urologic evaluation. Frightened by this symptom, men hope that the problem will go away by itself if they abandon sexual intercourse. This is foolhardy behavior. A visit to the doctor will help uncover the reason for the bloody semen. Often bladder or prostate infection, and occasionally prostate cancer, are responsible for the appearance of blood in the semen. Prompt treatment can be instituted, and then sexual function returns.

Does your partner enjoy sexual intercourse?

Sexual intercourse should be a shared pleasure. If the partner views sex only as an obligation and merely accommodates the man, then his pleasure will be diminished. For older women who have gone through menopause, sexual intercourse can be unpleasant. This is because the postmenopausal lack of estrogen hormones affects female sexual tissues, resulting in a narrowing or shrinking (atrophy) of the vaginal lining. Further, without estrogen, inadequate mucus is produced by the glands in the crypts of the vagina, and the vagina fails to lubricate normally, making intercourse painful. Treatments include local lubricating ointments or estrogen hormones. The advisability of either of these treatments should be discussed by the woman with her physician or gynecologist.

What form of contraception are you using?

For the younger woman, fear of pregnancy can be a major impediment to her continued enjoyment of sexual intercourse. Some women are likely to shy away from sexual activity unless they can be reassured that they will not become pregnant. A review of the couple's current contraceptive practices is in order. If fear of impregnation looms as a factor diminishing the enjoyment of sex, alternative contraceptive options should be considered.

Have you had any injury or inflammation of your testicles?

It is in the testicles that the hormone testosterone is manufactured and then released into the bloodstream. Adequate circulating testosterone levels are needed to maintain sex drive, or libido. If the testicles are injured or attacked by a virus, their capacity to generate sufficient testosterone may be diminished. Then serum testosterone levels and sex drive decline. Inflammation of the testis (orchitis is the medical term) is usually exquisitely painful and not readily dismissed. However, there are some more furtive forms of testicular inflammation that cause only a flulike illness with characteristic muscle aches and pains. In such cases the pain is often mistakenly identified as a groin muscle pain and considered merely an integral part of the flu.

When a virus invades the testicle it causes first a swelling and then a shrinkage in testicular volume. A man may be aware that his testicle is smaller then it used to be. Recollection of "normal" testicular size can be a perilous and slippery slope. The passage of years has a magnifying effect on our memory. In retrospect, the genital size of our youth seems to be more substantial than it actually was.

Are you having trouble sleeping?

Depressed, impotent men have difficulty sleeping (insomnia). They fall asleep readily but cannot stay asleep. They usually say they go to bed at about 11:00 P.M., then wake up in the middle of the night and are unable to fall back to sleep.

While it is true that older men frequently awaken in the middle of the night, they do so to urinate. Usually when they return to bed they fall asleep promptly. Depressed men do not. Recognition and treatment of the depression is a priority if sexual function is to return.

Routine questions regarding general health are now in order; issues of critical importance relate to a history of high blood pressure (hypertension), diabetes, heart disease, pelvic surgery or X-ray therapy, prescription medications, or other chemical use.

High blood pressure. Hypertension can impair male sexual function. Impotence is about three times as common in untreated hypertensive men than in men of similar age who have normal blood pressure. We are not sure why. Persistent high blood pressure possibly invites hardening and narrowing of the small blood vessels in the penis. When this occurs, blood cannot flow with the same freedom into the erectile bodies, making it difficult for people with hypertension to achieve or sustain erections.

Almost all men with high blood pressure are treated with antihypertensive medications, some of which have sexual side effects. (See Chapter 9, "Medications, Chemicals, and Potency.")

Diabetes mellitus. Impotence is a common problem for diabetic men. Sexual problems do not surface when diabetes first appears, but after some years the diabetic process can damage blood vessels and nerves needed for erections. The large or medium-size arteries become clogged, and blood cannot reach the penis with sufficient force to create an erection. Diabetes also can scar smaller arteries, restricting the "breathing room" of the penile erectile cylinders so they cannot expand sufficiently for a fully rigid erection.

Diabetes also disables the nerves that normally signal penile blood vessels to start trapping blood to hold an erection. Symptoms and signs of this diabetic nerve damage (neuropathy) include numbness or tingling of the legs and feet and difficulty in fully emptying the bladder.

Heart disease. During sex, heart rate and blood pressure increase. The heart requires additional oxygen. If the arteries leading to the heart are narrowed because of atherosclerosis (hardening of the arteries), they cannot provide a sufficient supply of oxygenated blood to accommodate those increased demands of the heart. When this occurs, a frightening chest pain, called angina pectoris, can develop. The pain acts as a powerful countervailing force to continued sexual activity. If a man has experienced such pain during sexual intercourse, his physician will want to schedule diagnostic studies to determine whether the pain is due to coronary artery disease or other problems.

The increase in heart rate and blood pressure during sex is so predictable that sexual activity can be thought of as a "stress test" that stretches the limits of cardiac reserve. But bear in mind that men who have had heart attacks and even those who have had cardiac surgery can, after a period of recuperation, return to a normal sex life. However, an appropriate amount of time must elapse to allow the damaged heart muscle to recover and surgical wounds to heal.

An extensive patient/doctor discussion of the wisdom of continued sexual activity is prudent. Then a collaborative decision to develop a plan for an appropriate and safe pace of physical activity leading to the resumption of sexual intercourse is sensible.

Surgery or X-ray treatment. Surgery, particularly in the lower abdomen, may restrict blood flow or neurologic signals needed for normal erections and ejaculation. Of specific interest is a history of vascular or arterial surgery that focuses on restoring blood flow to leg muscles without attending to a man's sexual needs. The aorta pumps blood to the lower extremities and pelvis. Blood cannot flow freely through blood vessels narrowed by atherosclerosis. This limits the supply of blood to the penis and legs (see chapter 7). Surgery intended to restore blood flow to the legs may result in inadvertent injury to the smaller blood vessels or nerves required for full erectile vigor.

Prostate surgery sometimes injures the systems required for normal forward ejaculation.

Malignancies that have spread to the lower abdomen are often treated with surgery or radiation therapy (X-ray treatment). Neurologic control of the systems responsible for normal erections is disabled by these treatments. This causes impotence or an inability to ejaculate.

Prescription medications. Several drugs, specifically antihypertensives and antidepressants, as well as those commonly used to treat ulcers, can impair sexual responsiveness. Frequently, an adjustment in medication type or dosage is all that is needed to restore sexual potency (see chapter 9).

Other chemical use. The chemicals in prescription medications are not the only substances responsible for disrupting male sexual function. Thus, the routine medical history contains questions concerning alcohol consumption, cigarette smoking, and use of marijuana, cocaine, and heroin. All these substances, when used in excess, can sabotage the operation of internal systems responsible for sex drive, erections, and ejaculation (see chapter 9).

The Physical Exam

After taking the medical history, the doctor will perform a physical exam. He or she will look for previously undiagnosed high blood pressure, diabetes, heart disease, and prostate problems. In addition, there are several unique features of the exam when sexual difficulties are involved.

Visual field exam. This test helps determine whether any loss of vision has occurred in the corner of the eyes. Pituitary tumors press on the portion of the eye nerves responsible for lateral or peripheral vision. They may also interfere with testosterone production, resulting in impotence.

Thyroid. The thyroid gland sits in the neck in front of the wind pipe (or trachea). The thyroid regulates virtually all the metabolic processes of the body and, when not functioning properly, can have a profound effect on desire and potency. The doctor can feel whether the thyroid is large or lumpy; patients whose impotence is caused by an over- or underactive thyroid (hyper- or hypothyroidism) have distortions in thyroid anatomy that can readily be detected.

Pulses. As noted, adequate blood flow to the penis is essential for normal erections to occur. The easiest way to evaluate blood flow is to feel a patient's pulse, particularly in the arteries in the groin and lower legs. Men with atherosclerosis or other problems that restrict blood flow have dampened pulses. If weak or absent pulses are found, blood flow to the genitals may also be inadequate.

Neurologic exam. Signs of nerve damage (neuropathy) can be detected by simple maneuvers. Decreased sensation to the touch of a feather or pinprick, or sluggish or absent knee and ankle reflexes suggest a defect in the nerves that normally carry sensation and activate reflexes.

Penis and testicles. The penis is checked for any firm, fibrous bands or distortions in shape that would indicate underlying Peyronie's disease (see page 31). Testicular size is estimated. A substantial variation exists. Nevertheless, testicles less than 3.5 centimeters (1½ inches) are considered small. Truly atrophied testicles appear as pea-size nubbins in the scrotum.

It is also important to determine whether both testicles have descended fully into the scrotum. Normally, the testicles descend immediately before birth. Some testicles do not complete the migration; they become nonfunctional and can produce neither adequate amounts of testosterone nor sperm.

The length of the penis is rarely a factor in sexual dysfunction. For the very few men whose erect penis is too small for penetration, reconstructive surgery is possible.

6

The Impulses for Potency:
The Nervous System

Not all erections are the same. Different parts of the nervous system are called into play to allow men to have spontaneous erections, erections after genital stimulation, and unstimulated nighttime or early-morning erections.

Spontaneous, or Psychogenic, Erections

So-called psychogenic erections orginate in response to stimuli that excite the senses. Specific sights, smells, sounds, nongenital touching, and even imagination may initiate a psychogenic erection. The brain perceives these sensations and then transmits nerve impulses to the thoracolumbar erection center in the spinal cord just below the lower chest (thorax) and just above the upper back (lumbar area). This site can provoke erections by signaling pelvic nerves to start the flow of blood into the penis.

Neurologic messages from the thoracolumbar erection center can also coordinate with a second erection center located in the lower back (sacral area), which can initiate or reinforce an erection by signaling to nerves in the pelvis.

Reflex Erections

Direct genital stimulation can also provoke an erectile response. This type of erection is referred to as a reflex erection because it can occur in the absence of erotic stimuli. It is, in a sense, the genital equivalent of a knee-jerk.

All of us have experienced a knee-jerk; when the doctor taps our knee with a little rubber reflex hammer, our leg automatically jerks forward. This is a classic example of a stimulus-response reflex. The tap of the hammer on the knee is the stimulus for the initiation of a nerve impulse that travels with lightning speed to a junction in the spinal cord. Here the reflex arc is completed as a second signal speeds down another nerve to make the leg muscle contract so that the leg kicks forward. The same basic principle can be used to understand how men acquire reflex erections.

Stroking of the scrotum and penis triggers neurologic signals in a local genital nerve called the pudendal nerve. The pudendal nerve then carries the message directly to the sacral erection center, which initiates the response by flashing a reflex impulse so that the erectile cylinders of the penis can fill with blood and the penis becomes erect.

During sex, men probably utilize both the psychogenic and reflex systems and take advantage of both the thoracolumbar and sacral erection centers.

Stimulating and Inhibiting Penile Erections

Until recently, researchers were stymied in their attempts to study the phenomenon of psychogenic erections. They have been obliged instead to rely on an examination of the factors responsible for the development and maintenance of reflex erections. Because they work through a reflex cycle activated by direct rather than indirect stimulation, reflex erections can be readily induced and studied.

Normally, reflex erections occur as couples engage in genital foreplay. Researchers have recruited men to participate in a study to determine exactly how reflex erections are achieved and sustained. Volunteer partners for the recruits, however, were not used. Instead, a mechanical vibrator was applied to the genital area.

Once initiated, a reflex erection can be sustained as long as the man is not burdened by any competing neurologic demands. A man who has been stimulated to a full reflex erection will promptly lose his erection when asked to do a nonsexual task such as mental arithmetic. When instructed to discontinue the task, he may respond to further genital stimulation to restore his erection; he can then augment his erection through fantasy. This implies that a reflex-stimulated erection can be enhanced with psychogenic input. Another competing signal to the nervous system, such as an electric shock, will cause the erection to vanish.

These studies demonstrate how readily reflex erections can be induced, lost, and regained. This information has practical take-home value. Impotent men commonly complain about loss of an erection during lovemaking. But if a man is capable of achieving and sustaining an erection in the first place, it is reasonable to presume that both neurologic signals and vascular blood flow into the penis are normal. This implies that his erection can be reactivated with the proper stimulus. Psychogenic and reflex erectile systems will allow rigid erections to return as long as there is no distracting or competing neurologic signal.

Nocturnal Erections

A good night's sleep is an involved process. Several predictable stages of sleep are recognized: We become drowsy; fall asleep; fall into a deeper sleep; become more readily rousable and then fall into a still deeper sleep; then wake. Each stage of sleep generates its own distinctive pattern of neurologic signals. We know from studies of sleeping subjects that characteristic shifts in the brain wave or electroencephalogram (EEG) patterns reliably mark each sleep stage. During REM (rapid eye movement) sleep, the eyes dart rapidly back and forth under the eyelids and the neuroreflexes responsible for spontaneous nocturnal erections are activated.

Interludes of REM sleep occur sporadically throughout the night; normal men have about four episodes nightly. Each interval of REM sleep heralds the development of a new nocturnal erection (see figure 3). In fact, the penis may remain erect for a total of two hours each night. Men are unaware of most of these episodes, recognizing only the REM sleep–stimulated erection they have in the morning. Because that erection disappears after they urinate, men assume that this erection is due to the accumulation of urine in the bladder. This is not the case, since urine collects in the bladder throughout the day without stimulating erections.

Nocturnal penile tumescence persists throughout life. However, in later years episodes may be dissociated from REM sleep. After the age of sixty, men acquire the ability to achieve nocturnal erections during both REM and non-REM sleep. The reason for this age-related shift in nocturnal erections has not been satisfactorily explained.

The erections acquired during sleep and after stimulation are generally sufficient to allow for vaginal penetration. However, the sexual act does not end with penetration. Ejaculation must occur.

Ejaculation

Ejaculation requires a completely different set of neurologic signals. Once again the spinal cord plays a pivotal role. During the earliest phase, in preparation for ejaculation, fluid released from the testicle, prostate, and seminal vesicles seeps into ducts that connect to the tube (urethra) in the middle of the penis. Later a second set of nerve impulses is recruited to initiate vigorous contractions of the muscles of the pelvic floor. It is this pattern of muscle contractions that propels stored semen out of the genital tract and through the urethra during orgasm.

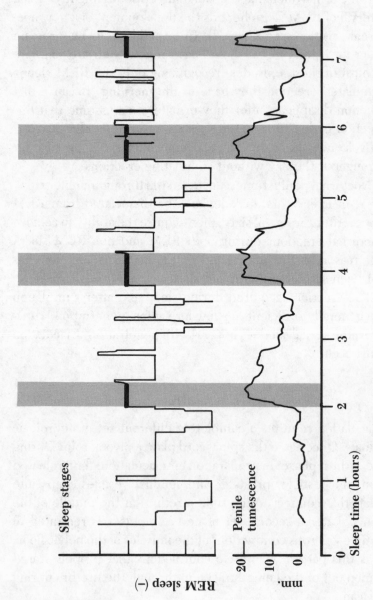

Figure 3. Nocturnal penile tumescence coincides with rapid-eye-movement (REM) sleep.

This elaborate neurologic circuitry is susceptible to different physical and chemical insults, which can interfere with the normal transmission of signals.

Specific Causes of Neurogenic Impotence

The very fact that disparate areas of the central and peripheral nervous system are vital for normal erection indicates that an equal number of sites are vulnerable to injury or malfunction. Impotence is the inevitable consequence of any condition that interrupts the normal flow of neurologic impulses in the brain, thoracolumbar erection center, sacral erection center, and peripheral nerves.

For purposes of discussion, it is convenient to compartmentalize neurologic problems causing impotence into those originating in the brain, the spinal cord, and the peripheral and autonomic nervous systems. (The peripheral nerves govern voluntary, the autonomic nerves involuntary, actions.)

The Brain

Temporal Lobe Epilepsy

Ordinarily, men with neurogenic impotence retain a normal sex drive. However, there is one group of men with a form of neurogenic impotence for whom the primary problem is a lack of sex drive. In their case, the loss of libido is caused by a type of epilepsy that originates in the temporal lobe of the brain. This condition is referred to as either temporal lobe epilepsy (TLE) or complex partial seizures. Unlike patients with conventional epilepsy, who suffer periods of unconsciousness and shaking, TLE patients have more subtle symptoms. They may experience periodic rage, occasional unexplained dizziness or fainting, auditory hallucinations, bed-wetting, and lapses of attention (called fugue states).

We are not entirely sure why only the epilepsy that arises

in the temporal lobe has such a devastating effect on sexual desire. Recently, researchers determined that a feedback loop exists between the temporal lobe and the hypothalamus, the area of the brain where signals critical for sexual function originate. The control of pituitary and ultimately testicular hormone secretion is dependent on hypothalamic signals. Epileptic discharges originating in the temporal lobe can disrupt normal hormone production.

For men with TLE, treatment of the hormonal abnormalities alone does not restore potency. Hormone treatment must be combined with conventional antiepilepsy medication (see chapter 8).

The Spinal Cord

Spinal cord injury at the thoracolumbar or sacral erection center causes a selective loss of erectile capability. Damage to the thoracolumbar erection center destroys the capacity for psychogenic erections. Men can no longer have erections merely by fantasizing or viewing sexually explicit material. However, they still can have reflex erections with genital stimulation. This is possible because reflex erections originate in the lower spine and use different nerve tracts from those required for psychogenic erections.

In contrast, men who have had lower spinal cord injury involving the sacral erection center lose the ability to have reflex erections. If their upper spinal cord remains intact, they can still have psychogenic erections.

Trauma severe enough to shatter the spine is caused by automobile and diving accidents, combat injuries, and gunshot wounds. These are among the most common disrupters of spinal cord impulses. The neurologic injuries caused by such violence produce profound defects in other nerve functions. Men with lower spinal cord injuries frequently lose the ability to move their legs. They may even lose the ability to empty their bladders. The spinal-cord-injured patient experiences a striking disruption in his daily life. Men with such severe neurologic impairment were until recently considered irrevocably impotent, and their sexual needs were ignored. A new generation has a more positive outlook.

Spinal cord injuries, although devastating, are not sexually fatal. The man who loses control of muscle function can still retain his interest in sex. He can be stimulated to some degree of erection, depending on the location of the injury. There is, as yet, no way to repair the nerve damage.

Ejaculation is more of a problem, but there are now means of stimulating ejaculation in a fashion similar to that used in animal husbandry. The electroejaculation techniques successful in collecting semen from breeding livestock have been used with some success in men. On rare occasions, patients with spinal cord injuries have been stimulated to ejaculate so that their semen could be collected and used to inseminate their partners.

In one large study of almost 1,300 men who had suffered spinal cord injury, 77 percent were able to have erections. Thirty-five percent engaged in sexual intercourse. Spontaneous ejaculation was possible in only 10 percent, however.

Lumbar Discs and Discogenic Impotence

Lumbar disc disease and sciatica are common medical conditions. The bones (or vertebrae) of the spinal column are separated from one another by cushions called intervertebral discs. These discs consist of a soft, gelatinous interior encased by tough, fibrous tissue. As long as the discs remain neatly stacked directly beneath the vertebrae, they cause no problem. But occasionally discs drift from their midline position and press on spinal nerves. If the disc presses on the sciatic nerve, the patient experiences pain down the side of his leg. Other nerves in the spinal cord are responsible for regulating bladder function and erections.

When the location of the disc interferes with a man's ability to have erections, he is said to have discogenic impotence. These men usually have other neurologic symptoms, such as lower back pain, difficulty ejaculating, occasional urinary dribbling, and pain radiating to their hips and down their legs.

Computerized axial tomography (CAT scan) reveals the location of a disc and its relation to the spinal cord; surgery frequently alleviates pain and corrects some of the urinary and sexual symptoms. But only about one-third of men with discogenic impotence experience a return of potency after the disc is removed.

Peripheral Nerves and the Autonomic Nervous System

Multiple Sclerosis

Multiple sclerosis (MS) is a poorly understood medical condition that can attack nerves throughout the body. The primary problem in MS is a loss of the normal protective sheath (or myelin) around nerves. Without this protective covering, nerves cannot transmit their messages coherently. When the nerves affected are in vulnerable areas of the spinal cord, impotence develops. Current estimates indicate that 50 percent of men with MS are impotent.

Multiple sclerosis is a chronic disease and given to inexplicable periods of sudden improvement (or remission) followed by deterioration (or exacerbation). When MS goes into a temporary remission, sexual function may return. But the course of the disease is capricious, and worsening may come just as suddenly and unpredictably. Therefore the sexual function of men with MS is always precarious and fluctuates over time. There is as yet no cure for this disease.

Syphilis

The bacteria that cause syphilis are called spirochetes. Because penicillin kills spirochetes, it was believed at one time that it would rid the world of the scourge of syphilis forever. Unfortunately, syphilis remains and has made a resurgence during the AIDS epidemic.

Men infected with syphilis first develop a hard ulcer on the tip or shaft of the penis. If this is ignored and syphilis remains untreated, the spirochete establishes a foothold and spreads to other organs. When syphilis invades the spinal cord, it destroys cells responsible for the neurologic reflexes that control erection and bladder sensation. Late-stage syphilis is treatable with penicillin, but spinal cord or neural damage is irreversible. Men in this late stage of syphilis cannot have erections or empty their bladders.

Diabetes Mellitus and Diabetic Neuropathy

As mentioned, diabetes mellitus is a common medical condition. It affects 10 million Americans, 4 million of them men. Diabetes sets in motion events that damage the heart, eyes, and kidneys and prevent nerves from transmitting impulses efficiently. The nerve damage is called diabetic neuropathy, and it takes several different forms.

Impotence in diabetic men may be a reflection of a neuropathy affecting several different types of nerves. Some nerves carry messages of sensation, like pain and pleasure. Others transmit impulses that allow the pelvic muscles to contract during ejaculation. One other critical component of the nervous system, the autonomic nervous system, is also vital for sexual function. The autonomic nervous system works silently and effortlessly and helps us get through many daily functions.

For example, in the morning, when we first stand up, our blood pressure drops. This fall is temporary; the autonomic nervous system instigates a battery of neural responses that helps stabilize blood pressure. Diabetic patients with autonomic neuropathy cannot do this. Because diabetes has damaged their autonomic nervous system, they cannot marshal a prompt increase in blood pressure. Diabetics' blood pressure often falls to very low levels, occasionally causing fainting.

The autonomic nervous system also plays an important role in transmitting messages for erections, ejaculation, and bladder function. Diabetic men with autonomic neuropathy become impotent, are unable to ejaculate, and may even have trouble emptying their bladders completely when they urinate.

Inadequate autonomic nervous system function can also occur in older nondiabetic men. Idiopathic autonomic insufficiency produces similar symptoms of inability to stand upright without feeling faint, loss of the ability to empty the bladder, impotence, and inability to ejaculate.

In terms of sexual potency, men with diabetes mellitus are twice cursed. In addition to causing nerve damage, diabetes attacks the blood vessels that must dilate and enlarge to pump blood into the penis for an erection to develop.

Symptoms suggesting diabetic nerve damage include loss of sensation at the tip of the penis, numbness of the lower extremities, and spasms or unexplained pain in the legs.

The regularity with which impotence occurs in diabetics is striking. Young diabetics have no more sexual dysfunction than their nondiabetic contemporaries. But they can anticipate a progressive decline in sexual function. Ten years after the onset, 50 percent of diabetic men will be impotent. By age seventy, more than 95 percent are impotent. We do not yet know how to repair diabetic nerve damage, although there are treatments for the impotence it causes. Penile implants (see chapter 12) and penile injections (see chapter 13) have been used to help restore potency in men suffering from diabetic neuropathy.

Chronic Kidney Disease

The kidney filters waste products from the bloodstream to be excreted in the urine. When the kidney can no longer accomplish this task, waste products build up in the bloodstream and cause a condition known as uremia. In the past, uremic men and women had a limited life expectancy, and sexual function was not a primary concern. However, with the availability of dialysis therapy and kidney transplants, life expectancy for uremic people has been greatly extended.

As chronic renal disease persists and dialysis becomes a way of life, two systems vital for normal male potency fail. For reasons that are still unclear, dialysis patients experience nerve damage. When this extends to the nerves required for normal erections, impotence develops.

Kidney disease can also disrupt the endocrine system. Production of testosterone declines, and secretion of prolactin, a sexually inhibiting hormone, increases. Low serum testosterone and high serum prolactin levels individually or together can cause impotence. Treatment aimed at normalizing serum prolactin and testosterone values can help restore sexual function.

Diagnosing Neurogenic Impotence

The number of tests currently used to evaluate neurologic function in impotent men is increasing. Many of the more sophisticated invasive tests are primarily investigational and are best performed in research centers. For the majority of men, the information provided by these tests is little more than the frosting on the diagnostic cake. Symptoms and signs of neurologic problems can usually be detected in the medical history and physical exam. For example, diabetic men with absent reflexes and diminished sensation in their lower extremities can be presumed to have nerve damage. If they also are impotent, it is reasonable, in the absence of other compelling information, to presume that nerve damage is the cause of the impotence.

Two general classes of neurologic tests are used in the evaluation of impotence. The most popular test, the nocturnal penile tumescence test, assesses the man's ability to achieve and sustain erections during the night. Other neurologic function tests evaluate the integrity of individual nerves responsible for reflex erections and ejaculation.

Tests of Nocturnal Penile Tumescence

The observation that normal men experience spontaneous erections during sleep has been common knowledge since the early 1950s, but this phenomenon was not studied in detail until 1965. In that year, Dr. Ismet Karacan, then a doctoral candidate in New York, introduced the scientific world to the concept of nocturnal penile tumescence (NPT) monitoring. Dr. Karacan knew that erections occurred during the particularly restful REM sleep. His pioneering studies and those that followed evolved from careful evaluations of normal men in hospital sleep laboratories. The men's brain wave patterns, eye movements, and number, strength, and duration of erections were recorded.

A device something like a blood pressure cuff is placed around the man's penis before he falls asleep. As erections develop, the swelling and enlargement of the penis create pressure, which is recorded and then studied with the pattern of brain waves and eye movements.

The NPT test is often used as the "definitive" diagnostic test to determine whether a sexually dysfunctional man has organic or psychogenic impotence. Men who do not have nighttime erections are classified as having organic impotence, whereas those who have a full complement of nighttime erections are diagnosed as having psychogenic impotence. But results from one night's testing are not always reliable. Often, repeat testing is necessary to establish validity of the diagnosis. This is expensive and not always covered by health insurance. Thus, alternative methods of NPT testing have been developed.

Snap Gauge

The snap gauge is fitted around the shaft of the limp penis at bedtime. The gauge is equipped with three bands of different tensile strength so that increasing amounts of penile enlargement are required to break each ring. Minor swelling will break only the first ring; further swelling will break the second ring; but only a fully rigid erection will rupture the third ring.

The snap gauge has the advantage of being relatively inexpensive and does provide limited information about erectile capability. It does not, however, provide any information on the nature and extent of REM sleep or the frequency and duration of nocturnal erections. A single brief (say, thirty-second) erection would break all three rings but would be inadequate for intercourse.

Rigi-Scan

Rigi-Scan is a new device calibrated to provide information on penile rigidity as well as swelling (tumescence). One of the problems still plaguing standard NPT tests, even those performed in sleep laboratories, is that recordings of tumescence do not provide information about rigidity. The Rigi-Scan seeks to correct that deficiency.

The Rigi-Scan is a portable instrument with a computer chip and two rings. One ring is affixed to the tip of the penis and the other to the base. The rings are attached in the doctor's office, and the patient wears the unit home. During sleep the nature and extent of his erections are recorded on a small disk in the unit. The patient returns in the morning, and the physician retrieves the disk and downloads it into a standard computer. Results of erectile activity and penile rigidity are generated back on the computer monitor.

Rigi-Scan units generate NPT results at a fraction of the cost of a laboratory sleep study done in a hospital. The Rigi-Scan also provides a convenient means of evaluation over several nights.

New Thinking about the NPT

Although many physicians still rely on NPT results to segregate impotent men into psychogenic and organic categories, others have challenged the basic premise of the NPT test.

What does it mean if a man has involuntary erections at night in a hospital but cannot have an erection when he attempts to have sex? Is there any way to evaluate the ability to achieve an erection in response to sexually provocative stimuli? Several investigators have attempted to refine the NPT test to do precisely that. They have developed techniques to compare results of spontaneous penile tumescence during sleep to the penile tumescence stimulated by erotic arousal.

This new approach requires a two-stage study. Standard NPT testing is done in one night in a sleep lab. On another day penile tumescence is measured as a man views a series of videotapes. A sexually neutral film, usually a travelogue, is followed by a tape depicting oral and genital heterosexual sex. In addition to the measurement of penile tumescence, subjects are asked to advance a lever to indicate how aroused they were by either film.

All men, potent or impotent, reported significant subjective arousal when viewing the erotic videotape. Some men considered to have psychogenic impotence had a normal complement of erections during the night and a normal complement of erections when viewing the erotic videotape. The diagnosis of psychogenic impotence seemed secure. Nevertheless, a susbstantial number of men who had spontaneous nocturnal erections and described the erotic videotape as arousing did not have an erection when viewing that film.

This discordant pattern of erectile responses helps fill in significant gaps in our knowledge. The NPT test, after all, provides information regarding the integrity of neurologic transmission and blood flow to the penis. If a man has an erection during the night, it is likely that he does not have neurogenic or vascular impairment. The addition of the erotic videotape should confirm the NPT results. But this turns out not to be the case. There now appears to be a subset of men originally thought to have psychological problems who may have spontaneous erections while they sleep but do not have erections in response to standard erotic stimuli. No matter how enticing or alluring their partner, the neurologic systems responsible for initiating psychogenic or reflex erections do not work. Possibly these men have a subtle malfunction in the system responsible for activation of these erections; we do not yet have the answer. But it is likely that a minor disruption in the way the brain receives and processes erotic material is responsible.

Other Neurologic Function Tests

Cremasteric Reflex

Stroke a man's inner thigh, and that side of his scrotum contracts. This is a cremasteric reflex. Stroking the thigh sends a signal to the thoracolumbar erection center, which then completes the reflex by transmitting a neural impulse to contract the scrotal muscle. This resembles what happens during a psychogenic erection. The reflex is absent in patients with diabetic neuropathy and multiple sclerosis.

The Scrotal Reflex

The scrotal reflex is less selective. Put any healthy man in a cold room and his entire scrotum will contract, bringing both testicles up toward the groin. The same reflex can be brought about by applying ice to the inner thigh. The scrotal reflex is absent in men with multiple sclerosis, though it is not clear how important it is in normal sexual function.

Bulbocavernosus Reflex Latency (BCRL) Time

The bulbocavernosus reflex time tests the integrity of nerve transmission. If the tip (glans) of the penis is squeezed, a neurologic signal will flow to a nerve in the lower spine to activate a reflex causing the muscles around the anus (the bulbocavernosus muscles) to contract. These muscles are called into play when a man ejaculates. The BCRL test measures the time it takes for an electrical stimulus applied to the tip of the penis to cause a contraction in the muscles surrounding the anus. Small needles with recording electrodes are placed in the muscle near the anus, and an electrical stimulus is applied to the tip of the penis—causing the patient brief, mild discomfort. The interval between the stimulus and the contraction is called the bulbocavernosus reflex latency (BCRL) time (see figure 4).

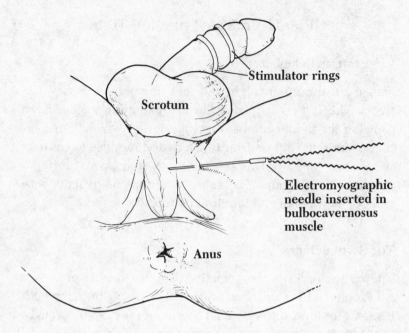

Figure 4.   Insertion of recording electrodes in bulbocavernosus muscle for BCRL test.

In normal men, the muscle twitch is detected thirty-five to forty milliseconds after the application of the stimulus. In patients with nerve damage, particularly those with diabetic neuropathy, the interval between stimulus and twitch is fifty to eighty milliseconds. These findings can be used to evaluate the velocity of other neurologic signals.

Penile Biothesiometry

Penile biothesiometry helps determine whether penile nerves responsible for appreciating sensation are functioning normally. A small instrument capable of vibrating at variable frequencies is placed along the shaft and tip of the penis. Increasing (but low) levels of vibration are applied, and the man informs the physician when he first senses vibration (humming) on his penis. Younger potent men can detect very subtle vibrations; older men appreciate vibrations only when they occur at considerably greater frequency. Penile biothesiometry is performed at only a handful of institutions and remains, for the most part, a research tool.

Dorsal Nerve Stimulation

Dorsal nerve stimulation is a variation on the BCRL theme. This test evaluates the nerves that carry signals from the penis to the spinal cord and then up to the brain. An electrical stimulus applied to the penis is first appreciated at the level of the spinal cord and only later in the brain. Norms for this test have been established in only a few groups of men. As might be anticipated, velocity of transmission along the dorsal nerve is slower in patients with nerve damage due to diabetes or alcoholism. The value of this test in the study of impotent men remains to be established.

Treatment of Neurogenic Impotence

Men with neurogenic impotence have three options. They can adopt a fatalistic view and live with their impotence, choose to have penile implant surgery, or learn to inject the drug papaverine into their penis to achieve an erection. Unfortunately, it is these men who are most susceptible to priapism, a prolonged painful erection, the most worrisome side effect of papaverine. The benefits and risks of penile injections as a treatment for impotence are reviewed in Chapter 13, "Penile Injection."

Prior to the introduction of this novel therapy, many men with neurogenic impotence relied on penile implants (or prostheses) as the only treatment that would provide the penis with sufficient rigidity for intercourse. Penile prostheses have been inserted with variable success. Impotent diabetic men have a higher rate of complications from such surgery than do men with other forms of neurogenic impotence. This is most likely because diabetic men are unusually prone to infection, and following surgery the development of an infection, especially in the area of the penile implant, can threaten the survival of the prosthesis. This is discussed in more detail in Chapter 12, "Penile Implants."

7

The Flow of Blood:
Arteries and Veins

The transformation of the penis from a limp to an erect state is an event requiring an unrestricted flow of blood into specialized cylinders in the penis (the corpora cavernosa and the corpus spongiosum). It is the unusual architecture of these cylinders that makes it possible for a man to develop an erection. The erectile tissue is in reality an elaborate spongy honeycomb designed to trap blood. In the early stages of an erection, blood is diverted into these spongy spaces. As they absorb more blood, the penis becomes fully erect. When a maximum erection is achieved, blood does not flow out of the penis because the draining veins are choked off (or compressed).

The penis remains erect until ejaculation. Then the spongy cylinders discharge their captured blood back into the bloodstream, and the penis reverts to its normal flaccid state. When the arterial inflow and venous outflow systems break down, vasculogenic impotence develops.

If a man's penile erectile cylinders do not fill with blood, he will be unable to initiate an erection. If blood trapped and stored in the penis leaks out prior to ejaculation, he will be unable to maintain his erection. Thus, vascular problems causing impotence have been defined as either "failure to fill" or "failure to store."

Failure to Fill

Blood released from the heart is pumped through arteries to provide oxygen to the heart as well as to the lungs, brain, kidney, and other tissues. The aorta is the main conduit for transfer of blood from the heart to the rest of the body. It can be thought of as a large tree with branches emerging at different junctions to supply blood to individual sectors of the body. The main branch bringing blood to the pelvis is the iliac artery. The iliac artery spawns its own subdivisions. Some branches supply blood to the lower extremities as well as the buttocks. Another tributary, the internal pudendal artery, is responsible for ferrying blood to the six small arteries nourishing the penis and its corporal erectile cylinder bodies (see figure 5). For most of the day, blood bypasses the erectile cylinders and serves only the needs of the penis.

To convert the penis from a limp to an erect organ, blood must first be diverted from the penile arteries into the erectile tissue through a series of small blood vessels called helicene arteries. Intrapenile vascular spaces called sinusoids start trapping blood during the early phases of penile swelling. When these sinusoids become sufficiently engorged, they swell and compress the surrounding veins to prevent blood from leaving the penis. As long as blood remains trapped within the corporal bodies under sufficient pressure, the penis stays erect (see figure 6).

Impotence due to a failure to fill is the result of sluggish blood flow to the penis. Problems restricting the flow of blood can originate at any level of the arterial tree; large, medium-size, and tiny arteries can be blocked.

When obstruction is present in a large artery, like the iliac artery, a limited amount of oxygenated blood is available for

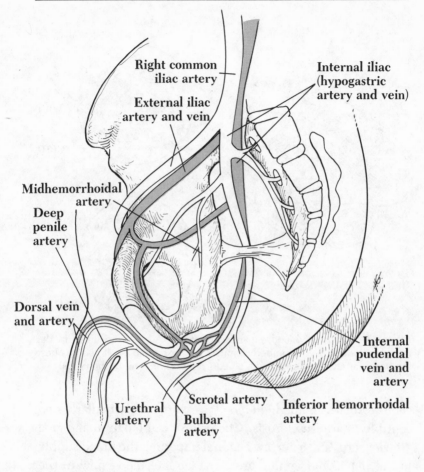

Figure 5.   Location of arteries supplying blood to the penis.

the muscles of the lower extremities as well as the pelvic arteries. In addition to impotence, symptoms reflecting the inadequate blood supply to the leg muscles are cramps in the calf muscles and leg pain after long walks. If, on the other hand, vascular disease is confined to the small blood vessels in and around the area of the penis and the sinusoids, impotence will be the only symptom.

Two basic problems, atherosclerosis (hardening of the arteries) and arteriolarsclerosis (scarring of the arteries), can restrict blood flow to the penile area. Men with high serum

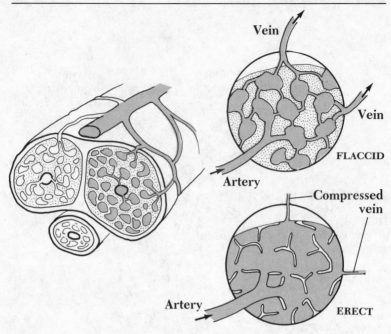

Figure 6.   Inflow of blood expands minute chambers (sinusoids) in the penile cylinders. The expanded chambers compress the small veins against the tunica albuginea, preventing blood from draining out of the penis.

cholesterol levels and high blood pressure are particularly susceptible to atherosclerosis. Cholesterol can lodge in and clog arteries, creating a narrow channel impeding the blood supply to the pelvis and genital area. Inadequate blood flow to the penile arteries prevents the full and uninterrupted transfer of blood into the penile erectile cylinders. Men who are heavy smokers or are diabetic often experience local arterial inflammation and scarring. This, too, restricts blood flow to the penis.

Some men are more likely than others to develop impotence due to a failure to fill. They can be recognized early in their adult life because of the presence of four arterial risk factors (ARFs): high blood pressure (hypertension), smoking, high serum cholesterol levels, and diabetes mellitus.

In one study, evidence of hypertension, diabetes mellitus, heavy cigarette smoking, or high cholesterol levels was found in 79 percent of men with failure to fill. The chance of developing this type of impotence increases as the number of ARFs mount up. The man with high blood pressure and high cholesterol levels who smokes has about a 50 percent chance of developing impotence due to a failure to fill as early as age fifty-five.

The number and type of ARFs also have implications for treatment options. For men suffering from atherosclerosis and selective narrowing of larger arteries due to high serum cholesterol levels and high blood pressure, the area of arterial obstruction can be removed or bypassed by a vascular surgeon so that blood flows more freely to the pelvis, allowing sexual function to be restored. Diabetic men and smokers are more likely to develop scarring of the small blood vessels in and around the penis. This is not amenable to surgery.

Symptoms

Impotence due to a failure to fill is a reflection of inadequate blood flow to the penis. Only rarely is this process confined to the arteries carrying blood to the genitals. An inadequate supply of oxygenated blood anywhere in the body creates its own set of distinctive symptoms.

Deprived of oxygen, the brain cannot think well, the kidneys stop making urine, and muscles cry out in pain. Angina pectoris is the term used to describe oxygen deprivation to the heart muscles. Claudication describes insufficient blood flow to other muscles.

Oxygen demand is activity dependent. A muscle at rest requires a minimal supply, whereas an active muscle demands a rich supply of oxygenated arterial blood. Muscles cramp when they do not receive adequate oxygen. This may be apparent only when the muscle is challenged by exercise.

Warren at age sixty-eight was no longer able to achieve an erection. He maintained that he was physically fit and cited as proof the fact that he played eighteen holes of golf two to three times a week. When pressed he did admit that his actual exercise was limited because a motorized golf cart, rather than his legs, was his source of transportation on the course. Only when he sliced a shot into the woods did he extend his exercise. Unfortunately, the last few times he prowled around the woods he developed such severe leg cramps that he was forced to sit down and rest. Symptoms of claudication reflecting inadequate blood flow became manifest only when Warren was forced to expand his range of activity.

Similar information can be obtained from nongolfers by simply asking them how far they actually walk each day and whether they can push themselves and extend that activity without experiencing any discomfort in their legs or buttocks.

When impotence and muscular cramps in the legs coincide, it is likely that an artery that supplies oxygenated blood to the legs and pelvis is obstructed. Men suffering from these obstructions not only experience an inability to achieve an erection, but also find that they cannot walk as far as they used to: Walking for any duration causes the muscles of their legs or buttocks to cramp. When the man notices the association between cramps and vigorous walking, he will gradually, almost imperceptibly, adjust his activity. Once he restricts his walking, leg cramps and pain no longer trouble him. When questioned, he can say honestly that he does not now have pain when he walks. A physician trying to make a diagnosis often must pursue this issue with some diligence.

Symptoms of claudication are invariably associated with extensive narrowing or obstruction in the major arterial supply of blood to the pelvis and lower extremities. More selective areas of narrowing do occur and produce their own unusual set of symptoms, such as the pelvic steal syndrome.

Pelvic Steal Syndrome

The pelvic steal syndrome (also called the iliac steal syndrome) is a consequence of the competition between muscles of the lower legs and the penis for a marginal blood supply. In such a competition, the penis is destined to lose.

A man with pelvic steal syndrome can acquire an erection. Problems develop after penetration. When he attempts to thrust his hips, the erection deflates. Increased activity of the pelvic and lower leg muscles creates a demand for additional oxygenated blood. First cramping in the buttocks and legs occurs, then, as blood is diverted away from the penis to the buttocks and legs, the erection fades.

Men with this sort of vasculogenic impotence usually have a significant narrowing in one or both iliac arteries—the major branches of the aorta that carry blood to the pelvis. Surgical reopening of the artery restores potency.

Medium-Size and Small Arteries

Injury to small arterial tributaries out of the main artery may cause impotence without compromising blood flow to the lower extremities. In this case, cholesterol deposits obstructing these penile arteries stifle penile blood flow.

It is easy to see how major pelvic injury, pelvic X rays, and injury to the penis can lead to vasculogenic impotence either by directly interrupting blood supply to the penis or by injuring the lining of the artery, which eventually encourages the accumulation of cholesterol. But less dramatic forms of pelvic trauma may also be responsible for impotence. Pressure on penile arteries and nerves sufficient to disrupt sexual function has been reported in men who are long-distance bicyclists and even those who use a stationary bicycle for exercise. A sensation of tightness or pain around the tip of the penis while bicycling is a premonitory symptom that blood flow to the penis is inadequate or the penile nerves are being unduly compressed.

This symptom of penile pain occurs in 10 to 50 percent of men who participate in long-distance bicycling. Bicycle-seat-induced pressure restricting penile blood flow has even been incriminated as a specific cause of impotence in men whose bicycling is restricted to a stationary bike. The height and positioning of the nose of the bicycle seat are critical in determining whether penile blood flow and local nerve transmission to the head of the penis are compromised. Frequently, blood flow is restored and pressure on genital nerves alleviated by simply adjusting the height of the bicycle seat. In normal men, bicycle-seat-induced decreases in penile artery blood flow are temporary; within thirty minutes normal blood flow is restored.

Failure to Store

If the flow of blood into the penile erectile cylinders is inadequate because of arterial (inflow) problems, the penis can swell but lacks sufficient internal pressure to choke off the veins responsible for draining blood away from the penis. This sequence of events is responsible for the partial erection experienced by many older men; it is still considered a failure-to-fill problem.

Other men, however, have adequate erections initially but cannot maintain them long enough for intercourse. The penis fills, swells with blood, and becomes erect. Then gradually it deflates due to a progressive flow of blood out of the penile erectile cylinders. Despite inflow that normally would be adequate, the blood-trapping mechanism is impaired and blood cannot be contained in the penis—even if the rate of arterial inflow is accelerated.

It remains unclear what causes this failure-to-store problem, but because the penile vein provides the only channel through which blood can leave the penis, the diagnosis of penile venous incompetence has found favor among urologists.

The amount of blood that must be transferred to the penis to create an erection in the first place is prodigious. Normal men acquire a firm erection when about two ounces of blood per hour are pumped with sufficient force into the penile erectile bodies. Impotent men with venous incompetence can achieve an erection, but only if twice as much blood is pumped into the penis. Nevertheless, they cannot sustain the erection even if the flow of blood is maintained at a rate of *four* ounces per hour.

Today we know much more about the factors that inhibit blood flow to the penis than the conditions responsible for premature drainage of blood. Researchers as yet have been unable to associate venous insufficiency elsewhere in the body with penile venous incompetence. Only a history of prompt acquisition and rapid loss of a rigid erection suggests a diagnosis of penile venous incompetence.

Diagnostic Tests

A diagnosis of vasculogenic impotence requires a demonstration that blood flow into or out of the penile erectile cylinders is not normal.

Doppler Ultrasound Recording

The arteries that bring blood to the penis, like arteries elsewhere in the body, emit a characteristic pulse. A machine called a Doppler ultrasound uses a process similar to sonar to measure the pulse wave with some accuracy. Blood flowing freely in the penile arteries produces a vigorous pulse pattern; restricted blood flow produces a sluggish pattern.

In addition to estimating the strength with which blood pulses through the arteries in the penis, physicians can make an actual measurement of penile artery blood pressure. Blood pressure is usually recorded in two phases. The first number (systolic) measures the pressure when the heart contracts and pumps blood into the arteries. The second number (diastolic) measures the pressure when the heart is at rest between contractions. (The Doppler ultrasound records only the systolic blood pressure.)

Penile systolic blood pressure must be related to the blood

pressure in the arm (brachial blood pressure). This relationship is the penile brachial index (PBI).

Normally, blood pressure in the penis is slightly lower than blood pressure in the arm. An evaluation of blood flow to the penis can be determined by comparing systolic penile artery blood pressure to brachial systolic blood pressure:

$$\text{PBI} = \frac{\text{penile systolic blood pressure}}{\text{brachial systolic blood pressure}}$$

A PBI of 0.9 or greater is considered normal; a PBI of 0.7 or less indicates compromised blood flow to the penis. PBI values between 0.7 and 0.9 fall into a gray zone, with lower values more strongly suggesting vascular problems.

Nocturnal Penile Tumescence

The measurement of a man's ability to achieve an erection during sleep is nocturnal penile tumescence (NPT) testing (see pages 57–60). An NPT test is often performed to evaluate the integrity of penile blood flow. Men with inadequate blood flow do not have a full complement of erections during sleep.

Pharmacologically Induced Erections

The muscle relaxant papaverine, when injected directly into the penis, causes a loosening or dilation of the smooth muscles around the tiny intrapenile blood vessels and allows an erection to occur by encouraging increased intrapenile blood flow. If no erection occurs, physicians assume that the tiny blood vessels in the penis are too scarred to relax and expand to allow an onrush of blood (failure to fill). If, on the other hand, a full erection is acquired but not sustained, consideration must be given to the diagnosis of failure to store.

The diagnostic intrapenile papaverine injection is given by the physician. He or she places a rubber band around the base of the penis to ensure that the papaverine will be confined to the penis. The physician then injects a small amount of papaverine into one of the erectile bodies (corpus cavernosum). Within minutes, the penis should start to swell and become erect. If the erection appears to be full and turgid, it is presumed that the patient does not have any impairment in arterial inflow to the penis.

When a papaverine injection does not stimulate an erection, a limitation of arterial blood flow is strongly suspected as the cause of impotence. If, on the other hand, the penis achieves some degree of swelling but not enough to qualify as a normal erection, the diagnosis of venous leakage can be considered.

Like papaverine, intrapenile prostaglandin E_1 injections have been used to segregate men with vasculogenic impotence from men with other forms of impotence. Men with vasculogenic impotence do not experience an erection following prostaglandin E_1 injections, whereas men with all other types of impotence do. It is possible that prostaglandin E_1 is more sensitive and specific than papaverine in identifying men with vasculogenic impotence.

Cavernosagram

The cavernosagram is a special X-ray study designed to supplement the information provided by the papaverine-induced artificial erection. It provides visual images of what's going on inside the penis during an erection. A special dye is injected into the body (corpus cavernosum) of the penis. The dye appears white on the black X-ray film. As long as the penis remains erect, the dye stays in the area of the corporal cylinders. In a man with venous incompetence, the dye disappears rapidly through venous channels despite continued administration.

The cavernosagram can also help pinpoint the location of specific leaky veins. As such, it provides valuable preoperative information for the surgeon repairing the blood vessels.

Arteriography

Arteriography is a specialized X ray used to define the anatomy of arteries transporting blood to the penis. An artery in the groin is punctured with a hollow needle. A small plastic tube (catheter) is threaded through the hollow of the needle and then pointed in the direction of arteries that supply blood to the pelvic area. X-ray dye injected through the catheter travels down the arteries to provide a graphic illustration of how arteries look as blood (dye) flows to the pelvis and penile erectile cylinders. Arteriography locates the site or sites of arterial blockage, narrowing, or damage for the surgeon.

Treatment of Vasculogenic Impotence

Impotence due to a failure to fill is treated by isolating and identifying the site or sites obstructing the vigorous flow of blood to the penis. Vascular surgeons have become remarkably successful in creating new channels in arteries or bypassing areas of obstruction so that free flow of blood to the pelvic arteries can be reestablished.

The best surgical results have been achieved in men with well-defined narrowing in large or medium-size arteries. The surgeon removes the area or areas of obstruction and establishes a new, wide channel to restore a full flow of blood to the penis.

Surgery is successful in about one-third of the cases. Unfortunately, in about half of these men, the success is temporary. Impotence returns in six months to a year. In addition, another one-third experience postoperative priapism (persistent painful erections).

Failure to store requires a different approach. Several different methods have been devised to enhance the competence and holding capacity of the intrapenile veins so that they do not allow blood to drain prematurely from the penis during an erection. Sagging veins responsible for venous inadequacy are shored up by urologic surgeons. Sometimes the penile veins are closed or removed to limit the number of channels draining blood.

About 22 percent of men who have venous surgery experience immediate and sustained restoration of potency. About 19 percent remain impotent. An intermediate group of men (15 percent) experience a temporary restoration of potency. The remaining men (44 percent) can achieve an erection with intrapenile papaverine injections. Whether this response is sustained, or if men are willing to continue with a penile injection program, has not been reported (see chapter 13).

The reason for the disappointing results of venous surgery is not entirely clear. It is possible that current diagnostic tests lack specificity. Venous insufficiency may be only one factor responsible for sexual dysfunction. One urologist has found that the vast majority of impotent men who have venous insufficiency also have arterial inflow problems. Thus, correction of the venous leakage alone is unlikely to help.

This finding has prompted some urologists to combine arterial and penile venous surgery. Opening and widening the arterial channels bringing blood to the penis while simultaneously closing veins taking blood away from the penis has intrinsic appeal. Initial results have been promising, but it is still too early to know whether this dual surgical approach will be effective in the long term.

Dramatic improvements in sexual potency are apparent in some men following arterial or venous surgery. For many of them, potency is sustained. For men who experience only a temporary improvement in sexual function, the fault may lie in persistence of high blood pressure, smoking, and other arterial risk factors that allow vascular disease to redevelop and obstruct blood flow to the penis.

8

Hormones Regulate
Male Sexual Function

Hormones course through our bloodstreams every moment of every day, yet we remain oblivious to their presence. Only when production exceeds or fails to keep pace with our daily needs are we obliged to acknowledge the existence of hormones. Some hormones enhance, and others inhibit, normal male sexual function.

The word *hormone* comes from the Greek word *horman*, which means to "urge on." Testosterone is the hormone responsible for urging on man's sexual function.

Testosterone and Normal Male Sexual Function

Three critical functions of testosterone are:

- development of normal male genital anatomy
- activation and maintenance of adult male sex drive
- preservation of normal sperm production and fertility

The impact of testosterone is apparent very early in life.

Immediately before conception a swarm of sperm circle the ovum. Only one will inseminate. All others will be rebuffed. If the inseminating sperm carries a Y chromosome, the fetus will be genetically programmed to develop as a boy. The rest is up to testosterone. By the twelfth week of pregnancy, the fetal testicle begins to secrete testosterone. Testosterone and its metabolic offspring, the hormone dihydrotestosterone, help shape the appearance of the normal baby boy's genitals. The period of fetal testosterone production is brief, from the twelfth to the twenty-fourth week of pregnancy. After the twenty-fourth week of pregnancy, the testicle enters a state of hormonal hibernation and is dormant. By this time, the fleeting intrauterine exposure to testosterone and dihydrotestosterone has properly defined the genital anatomy of the male fetus.

Activation of Male Sexual Desire

At about age thirteen or fourteen, an extraordinary event occurs. The dormant testicle suddenly starts manufacturing testosterone again and releases large amounts into the bloodstream. This surge of testosterone provokes a series of dramatic and well-recognized events.

Glands in the skin increase the production of sebum; acne often follows. The vocal cords thicken; the voice first cracks, then deepens. Muscles grow. A midadolescent growth spurt occurs (at about age seventeen or eighteen, the bone growth centers close, signaling that the young man has attained his full adult height). Mustache and beard begin to appear. His sweat glands pump out secretions with a distinctly musky odor. Perhaps most remarkable, the penis becomes longer and wider, and the scrotum acquires wrinkled ridges. His testicles enlarge to fill the scrotal sac. He may note, for the first time, that he is starting to experience a stiffening of his penis in the middle of the night. This is the onset of nocturnal erections. He may also be befuddled to discover that he has had a nocturnal emission, or "wet dream." Equally perplexing is the sudden shift in attitude toward the girls in his class who are, inexplicably, no longer insufferable but actually desirable.

All these startling transformations are due to the hormone testosterone. Tethered and restrained during his preteen years, testosterone production is quite suddenly cut loose and set free to wreak havoc with his body.

What causes the sudden increase in testosterone production during adolescence?

Spontaneous testosterone secretion does not occur. The testicle requires a go-ahead signal from the pituitary gland to start producing testosterone. The pituitary hormone responsible for overseeing testosterone production is luteinizing hormone (LH). Under the influence of LH, the testicle starts siphoning cholesterol from the bloodstream. Enzymes in the testicle gnaw away at the unwieldy cholesterol molecule to manufacture and release testosterone.

Testosterone ushers in the anatomical modifications required for sexual and reproductive competence. Men require testosterone to maintain their sex drive and potency.

Anything that interferes with normal testosterone production or action causes a decrease in libido and ultimately impotence. Some men have suboptimal testosterone production as a consequence of inadequate pituitary stimulation of the testicle. Without LH to stimulate it, the testicle does not manufacture testosterone. But it is not only the mere availability of LH but also the manner in which LH is delivered that determines the testicle's ability to make testosterone.

The testicle is finicky. It will not respond to a steady stream of LH; it produces testosterone only when periodic bursts or pulses of LH appear in the bloodstream. This is precisely what occurs at the onset of adolescence when there is a sudden shift in activity in the hypothalamus.

The hypothalmus, pituitary, and testicle remain in a state of suspended animation until adolescence. Then, for reasons not fully understood, the hypothalamus acquires the ability to release bursts of a hormone that triggers the pulsatile secretion of pituitary LH. Pulses of LH released from the pituitary travel through the bloodstream to activate testosterone production.

LH is referred to as a gonadotropin because it stimulates the male gonad (testicle). The hypothalamic hormone, called gonadotropin releasing hormone (GnRH), provides the hypothalamic stimulus for pulsatile release of LH from the pituitary.

The hormonal interaction among the hypothalamus, the pituitary, and the testicles is a bond that persists throughout a man's life. This entire system, referred to as the hypothalamic-pituitary-testicular axis, is responsible for creating and maintaining potency and fertility (see figure 7).

Sperm Maturation and Fertility

Male fertility demands an output of hundreds of millions of sperm every day. Two hormones—testosterone and a second pituitary gonadotropin, known as follicle stimulating hormone (FSH)—are charged with the responsibility of ensuring that the testicle meets its daily quota for sperm production. FSH is released from the pituitary in tandem with LH in response to episodic pulses of GnRH. Both gonadotropins speed through the body to activate designated cells in the testicle.

FSH affects sperm production, whereas LH initiates testosterone production. The testosterone is required for sperm to mature and attain full fertilizing capability (see chapter 15).

Specific Hormone Problems

Low Testosterone Production

If a man loses his ability to maintain adequate testosterone production, blood testosterone levels will decline and he will suffer a diminution in sex drive and become impotent.

Conditions responsible for low testosterone output are designated as primary hypogonadism and secondary hypogonadism. When the testicle itself does not function properly, the

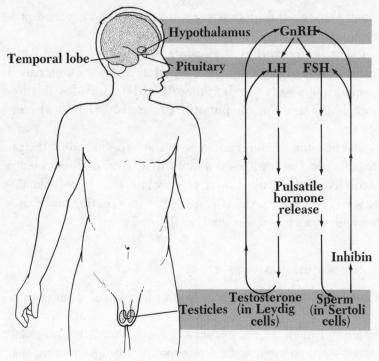

Figure 7.   Hormonal regulation of male sexual function.

diagnosis is primary hypogonadism. Secondary hypogonadism occurs when normal testicles cannot manufacture testosterone because the stimulating hormones of the pituitary or hypothalamus are missing or inadequate.

Primary Hypogonadism

Primary hypogonadism may be congenital (present at birth), acquired as the result of a virus that lodges in the testicles, or caused by external assaults such as testicular injury, radiation treatment, and chemotherapy.

Klinefelter's syndrome. Occasionally, failure of the gonads is ordained at conception. Instead of the normal complement of forty-six chromosomes, some men are born with one extra X chromosome. This results in an unusual chromosomal pattern—47 XXY instead of 46 XY. The condition is called Klinefelter's syndrome, after the physician who first recognized and described the characteristic physical features of this disorder.

Boys with the 47 XXY group of chromosomes are indistinguishable from other boys. The first signs of Klinefelter's syndrome surface during adolescence. The normal pulsating rhythms of the hypothalamus and pituitary start on schedule, but the testicles of the boy afflicted with this syndrome are unable to respond.

Some youngsters with Klinefelter's syndrome produce no testosterone at all. They retain a youthful appearance, but without testosterone to signal an end to their adolescent growth spurt they continue to grow and often become very tall. Under the continuous influence of growth hormone, boys grow taller, tower over their classmates, and often bring a twinkle to the eye of the high school basketball coach. Despite their height, young boys with Klinefelter's syndrome do not make good basketball players because their muscles remain unstimulated and undeveloped. This is yet another legacy of their testosterone deficiency.

Not all young men with Klinefelter's have such severe defects. Some boys make some testosterone early in their adolescence, do not grow to unusual heights, and become virilized. Their testicles produce testosterone briefly, then sputter, and thereafter fail. Men with the milder form of Klinefelter's syndrome have low sexual desire but may enjoy brief intervals of potency. They eventually suffer the same fate as their more severely affected counterparts. As their testicles fail, testosterone and sperm production cannot proceed and they are left impotent and infertile.

Mumps and other viruses. The cells that produce testosterone contribute very little to testicular size. Sperm-producing cells make up the bulk of testicular tissue. Often the same process that destroys the testicle's testosterone-producing capability also attacks the sperm-producing cells. When this happens, the testicle shrinks (or atrophies). This is often the fate of men who develop mumps as adults.

Childhood mumps generally spares the testicle. But when mumps strikes the adult male, the virus may spread through the bloodstream and attack the testicles. Initially the testicles swell and feel extremely tender. As the infection subsides, the testicles decrease in size. What follows is a predictable sequence of events. First sperm-producing, and later testosterone-secreting cells are damaged, compromising fertility and eventually sex drive and potency.

Raymond had two children, both in their twenties, both adopted. He had come to terms with his infertility and even joked that his low sperm count allowed him to save a fortune on birth control. Now, at fifty-seven, Raymond was impotent, and he had run out of jokes. The cause of his current impotence and prior infertility were traced to a common event. Thirty years earlier, while an elementary school teacher, he contracted mumps, which caused pain and swelling in both testicles. The pain was so severe that he could not bear to have his testicles touched and was obliged to wear an athletic supporter for two weeks. He and his wife resumed normal sexual activity when the swelling subsided, but she did not become pregnant. A semen analysis revealed that he had a low sperm count. That was when he and his wife decided to adopt. He remained potent for more than two decades. Then he noticed a gradual decline in his interest in sex and ability to acquire and sustain an erection. Hormone studies now revealed low serum testosterone levels. The infection that had destroyed his testicles' sperm-producing cells had left sufficient residual damage to compromise testosterone secretion. Testosterone treatment restored potency.

Other viruses that lodge in the testicles produce symptoms which are less dramatic than those of mumps, but the net effect is the same.

Secondary Hypogonadism

Men with normal testicles may still be incapable of producing testosterone if the stimulus to testosterone production is absent or blunted. The causes of secondary hypogonadism include benign tumors (or adenomas) of the pituitary and the hypothalamus.

Pituitary adenomas. The pituitary gland is responsible for regulating thyroid, adrenal, and testicular hormone secretion. When the pituitary becomes tumorous, this function cannot be sustained. It is still capable of low-level hormone production, but it cannot respond adequately to the pulsating hypothalamic GnRH hormone. As a result, pituitary hormones seep out, rather than burst out, into the bloodstream. The testicle will not respond to pituitary LH if it is not delivered in pulsatile bursts. Without LH pulses, the testicle cannot manufacture sufficient testosterone, and blood testosterone levels decline.

Tumors that destroy the pituitary's LH-secreting capability can also compromise other pituitary functions. It is in the pituitary gland that adrenocorticotropin (ACTH) and thyroid stimulating hormone (TSH) are made and released into the bloodstream to activate adrenal and thyroid hormone secretion, respectively. Inadequate secretion of all pituitary hormones causes a severe illness, panhypopituitarism. In addition to impotence, patients suffer low blood pressure, weakness, fatigue, and other symptoms of adrenal and thyroid hormone deficiency. The majority of these symptoms are relieved by adrenal and thyroid hormone medications. But treatment with testosterone restores potency to only 50 percent of the affected men; those who remain impotent have pituitary tumors that produce excessive amounts of the hormone prolactin. A study showed that men with pituitary tumors who regained potency with testosterone injections had low serum prolactin levels. Those who remained impotent had high serum prolactin levels (hyperprolactinemia).

We frankly do not know why men have prolactin-producing capability at all. Prolactin serves an important function in women, but only at a specific moment in their reproductive lives. At the end of a woman's pregnancy her pituitary produces and releases generous amounts of prolactin into the bloodstream to stimulate breast milk production. Nursing mothers usually have no menstrual periods because prolactin levels, when elevated, extinguish the pulses of pituitary hormones required to activate the normal menstrual cycle. When a woman stops nursing, prolactin levels decrease, pulsatile pituitary hormone secretion resumes, and menstrual function returns.

How does this relate to impotence in men? The same hormonal process that causes women to stop menstruating while they are nursing causes men to become impotent.

Hyperprolactinemia creates two problems that are inimical to sexual potency. Elevated serum prolactin levels inhibit normal pulsatile GnRH and LH secretion. The testicle is stranded without adequate stimulation and cannot produce its full ration of testosterone. Serum testosterone levels then fall. But giving more testosterone is not the remedy because elevated serum prolactin levels also prevent the body from responding normally to testosterone.

Two treatments—one surgical, the other medical—curtail excessive prolactin secretion by the pituitary.

Surgical removal of the prolactin-secreting pituitary tumor eliminates the source of excessive prolactin. Unfortunately, excision of only the pituitary tumor, while desirable, is not always feasible. Whittling away at the pituitary mass does make a significant dent in prolactin secretion, but rarely decreases it to the normal range. In these cases, impotence persists.

Doctors have discovered that a chemical in the body called dopamine normally reins in pituitary prolactin secretion in men. Without dopamine, prolactin levels increase. A selective dopamine deficiency in the hypothalamus is therefore presumed to be responsible for hyperprolactinemia in men. By restoring dopamine levels to normal, pituitary prolactin production is suppressed.

Bromocriptine (Parlodel), a medication with dopaminelike properties, is an effective dopamine surrogate. When hyperprolactinemic patients are treated with bromocriptine, serum prolactin levels usually return to normal within four to six hours. Continued treatment is required to keep prolactin levels fully suppressed.

Bromocriptine treatment has been effective in two regards. By lowering serum prolactin levels to normal, it restores sensitivity to the sexual effects of testosterone. Bromocriptine treatment also allows pulsatile pituitary hormone stimulation of the testicles to resume. As serum prolactin levels fall, serum testosterone levels increase and potency returns. Bromocriptine treatment also decreases pituitary tumor size and shrinks prolactin-secreting tumor tissue.

In some impotent hyperprolactinemic men, bromocriptine treatment alone suffices. Men with recent onset of impotence and small pituitary tumors are more likely to respond. Other men, especially those with large pituitary tumors, are not able to revitalize their own testosterone-producing capability without the additional help of testosterone injections. Once serum prolactin levels are normalized, these impotent men regain their responsiveness to the sexually stimulating effects of injected testosterone.

William was forty-one, weak, fatigued, impotent, about to lose his business and maybe his wife. His doctor noted that William had unusually low blood pressure and small testicles. X rays disclosed an enlarged pituitary, and blood tests established that—as a consequence of inadequate stimulation from his pituitary—adrenal, thyroid, and testicular production was subnormal. Treatment with adrenal and thyroid hormones so invigorated William that he was able to return to work, and his business prospered. Testosterone injections normalized serum testosterone levels, but he remained impotent. Ordinarily, testosterone-deficient men experience a brisk increase in sexual desire and potency with testosterone therapy. Treatment failures occur in men who have, in addition to their testosterone deficiency, other problems such as neuropathy, vascular disease, depression, or hyperprolactinemia. In William's case, hyperprolactinemia was the culprit. His large pituitary gland, incapable of supporting the function of his adrenal, thyroid, or testicle, was not totally inert, for it continued to produce prolactin in exorbitant amounts. Only when bromocriptine treatment normalized serum prolactin levels were testosterone injections effective in restoring William's sexual drive and potency.

Pituitary tumors are not the only causes of hyperprolactinemia. Many drugs used to treat high blood pressure, emotional problems, and gastric problems can compromise the action of dopamine and allow prolactin levels to increase. These include reserpine (Serpasil), methyldopa (Aldomet), chlorpromazine (Thorazine), trifluoperazine (Stelazine), thioridazine (Mellaril), haloperidol (Haldol), metoclopramide (Reglan), and prochlorperazine (Compazine).

Tumors of the Hypothalamus

Although the hormones responsible for triggering testicular hormone secretions are based in the pituitary, hormones released by the hypothalamus govern the fate of these pituitary hormones. Tumors of the hypothalamus severely limit the pulsatile release of hormones.

Hormone pulses must occur with sufficient frequency and reach sufficient amplitude to be effective. If the pulses occur infrequently, or with too little vigor, testosterone levels fall and men become impotent.

Time takes a toll on the intensity of the hypothalamic-pituitary signal to the testicle. (With aging, the hypothalamus slows down and pulses with less strength. But there is still enough testosterone to allow most older men to remain potent.)

Hypogonadism, Cause Unknown

One group of men with no visible hypothalamic or pituitary abnormality is incapable of launching pulsatile GnRH secretion at adolescence. Their LH pulses are totally absent, causing impotence and infertility. The condition, called idiopathic hypogonadotropic hypogonadism, can be corrected by reinstituting normal GnRH pulses.

Thyroid Hormone Disorders

The thyroid hormone thyroxine stabilizes the body's metabolism and allows us to proceed on an even keel from day to day. Both excessive and inadequate thyroxine production (hyperthyroidism and hypothyroidism) can interfere with normal male sexual function.

The diagnosis of thyroid hormone disorders is usually not difficult in young men. Nervousness, palpitations, weight loss, tremor, and anxiety are manifestations of excessive thyroid hormone secretion. Fatigue, lethargy, slowness of thought, constipation, dry skin, cold intolerance, and a deepening voice are indications of hypothyroidism.

In the older man, symptoms are more subtle. An irregular heartbeat or unexplained weight loss may be a clue to an overactive thyroid. Memory loss can reflect inadequate thyroid production. In the middle-age or older male, impotence may be the only obvious evidence of either condition.

Daniel, a fifty-two-year-old scientist, became impotent shortly after his divorce. His impotence was thought to be related to depression, and he had been seeing a psychiatrist for about one year. He had made some progress coping with his postdivorce depression, but his impotence persisted. Now he had a new problem—his left breast seemed to be growing.

Physical examination revealed a rapid pulse and a slightly enlarged thyroid. Daniel's left breast was indeed large and glandular. His hands trembled. The thyroid enlargement, increased breast size, rapid pulse, and tremor suggested the possibility of an overactive thyroid. Blood tests provided confirmation. With treatment, thyroid hormone levels normalized, breast tissue receded, and potency was restored.

Disorders of thyroid function are generally not considered in the evaluation of impotence despite the fact that loss of libido (in about 70 percent of cases), impotence (in about 55 percent of cases), and breast enlargement (incidence unknown) are prominent in hyperthyroid men. It remains unclear exactly how hyperthyroidism predisposes men to these sexual problems. The hyperthyroid state does create several associated hormonal abnormalities. Testosterone production is adequate, but the body converts an inordinate amount of the testosterone into an estrogen hormone (estradiol). Correction of the hyperthyroidism diminishes the stimulus for excessive estrogen production and coincides with a return of libido and potency.

Men with underactive thyroids tend to have low serum testosterone levels. Correction of the hypothyroidism usually allows serum testosterone levels to return to normal, and sexual function resumes. Unfortunately, some hypothyroid patients experience failure of both thyroid and testicular hormone secretion. For those men, treatment with thyroid hormone and testosterone together is necessary to restore metabolic, and then sexual, health.

Men with hypothyroidism have one other hormone abnormality that contributes to their sexual dysfunction. Their serum prolactin levels are often elevated. For them, bromocriptine treatment is unnecessary; thyroid hormone alone will normalize prolactin levels. Once prolactin levels normalize, sexual function resumes.

Treatments That Increase Testosterone Levels

Hormone therapy returns sexual function to the vast majority of men with hormonal abnormalities. The basic principle of any hormone therapy is to re-create a state of hormonal equilibrium. For men with thyroid or adrenal hormone disorders, this can be accomplished with hormone pills. Unfortunately, such is not the case for impotent men with testosterone deficiency.

Testosterone pills are available, but they are less effective than testosterone given by injection. Testosterone pills are not well absorbed from the stomach, and blood testosterone does not reach therapeutic levels. The pills also have a serious side effect: liver damage.

Once-a-month testosterone injections, although effective,

cause wide fluctuations in serum testosterone levels, with highest values occurring shortly after injection. Then, with normal metabolism, levels fall until the next injection. This results in a variable sexual response. Adjusting the dose or frequency of testosterone injections smooths out testosterone levels and maintains a steady state of sexual function.

Recently, an ingenious method for testosterone administration has been developed—the testosterone-impregnated skin patch. The patch is affixed to the thin skin of the scrotum, and the body absorbs a constant supply of testosterone. The patient simply changes the patch daily. This form of delivery may supplant injections as a means of normalizing circulating blood testosterone levels. The patch is still being studied but should be available shortly.

Three techniques, one old and two new, have been developed to allow men to increase the testosterone output of their own testicles.

As discussed, the testicles of men with secondary hypogonadism are normal but lack the appropriate pituitary stimulus to make testosterone. If that stimulus can be provided, the testicles should be able to function once again.

The older, traditional method takes advantage of a hormonal fluke. A hormone produced by women during pregnancy, called human chorionic gonadotropin (hCG), is an LH surrogate and acts directly on testicular Leydig cells to stimulate testosterone production. Synthetic hCG is available and when injected into the shoulder enters the bloodstream and provokes a brisk increase in serum testosterone levels. Unfortunately, the effect of a single hCG injection is short lived; twice-weekly injections are needed. This is more troublesome than a testosterone injection once a month. Today hCG treatment is reserved for infertile men with low sperm counts.

HCG acts directly on the testicle, bypassing the hypothalamus and pituitary. The two new treatment methods increase testosterone production by activating a man's own hypothalamus or pituitary.

Dr. William Crowley of the Massachusetts General Hospital has developed a small battery-powered pump that is loaded with the hypothalamic hormone GnRH. The patient wears the device on his hip. A thin tube extending from the pump ends in a needle that is placed under the skin of impotent men with GnRH deficiency (idiopathic hypogonadotropic hypogonadism). The pump is programmed to release pulses of GnRH to stimulate pulsatile pituitary LH release. Exposed to LH pulses, the testicle starts manufacturing testosterone and potency is restored. Pulsatile FSH release is also activated so that sperm production increases gradually. This enables a group of men previously thought to be hopelessly infertile to become fathers (see chapter 15).

Clomiphene, a medication commonly used to treat infertile women, can also stimulate testosterone production in some men with secondary hypogonadism. Clomiphene is effective in men because it increases pituitary LH and FSH stimulation of the testicle. Early pilot studies have been encouraging. One clomiphene tablet every other day can maintain normal testosterone levels. This avoids the peaks and valleys of blood testosterone values resulting from testosterone injections. Clomiphene therapy is still investigational and is approved only for the treatment of infertility in women.

Finding Hormone Problems in Impotent Men

All the necessary hormone measurements can be performed on the serum from one blood sample. Serum hormone levels normally vary throughout the day but generally fall within a range that is bracketed by an upper and lower limit called the reference range. When a man's blood hormone levels fall within the reference range, physician and patient can safely assume that sexual dysfunction is due to some other problem.

Hormone values do have a tendency to bob up and down throughout the day. Bear in mind: Slight increases in serum prolactin levels above, and modest decreases in testosterone below, the accepted ranges may occur in perfectly normal potent men. Men whose impotence is truly caused by disorders of hormone production have sustained and persistently subnormal blood testosterone, elevated prolactin levels, or abnormal thyroid hormone levels.

Physicians should routinely measure serum testosterone and prolactin values in impotent patients; thyroid hormone evaluation is usually reserved for those men who have symptoms or show physical signs compatible with disordered thyroid function.

How Common Are Hormone Problems in Impotent Men?

Hormone abnormalities, once thought to be a rare cause of impotence, are now recognized with increasing frequency. In one study of 422 impotent men at a Veterans Administration hospital, disorders of hormone secretion were detected in 29 percent. Primary hypogonadism and secondary hypogonadism dominated (19 percent), while 4 percent had hyperprolactinemia and 6 percent had disorders of thyroid hormone production.

This coincided with our prior experience. In a study of 135 impotent men, evidence of hormone dysfunction was found in 34 percent. We tended to see more hyperprolactinemic patients than our colleagues at the Veterans Administration.

A 1989 survey evaluated hormone function in 600 impotent men in Florida. Thirty-two percent (192 of 600) were found to have disorders of hormone secretion including testosterone deficiency (26 percent), hypothyroidism (6 percent), and hyperprolactinemia (3 percent).

Who Benefits from Hormone Therapy?

Hormone treatment is effective only in impotent men with bona fide hormone abnormalities. Indiscriminate use of testosterone, bromocriptine, or thyroid hormone is neither warranted nor effective; the practice of arbitrary administration of testosterone therapy to "boost" testosterone levels is similarly of no value. Testosterone increases libido and improves erectile function only in men with proven low testosterone production.

Adverse side effects of hormone therapy are uncommon. Muscular discomfort from an injection can be minimized by rotating the site of injection. Concern that repeated administration of testosterone might stimulate prostate growth or cancer in testosterone-deficient men has not proved to be a problem.

Bromocriptine can cause nausea and lightheadedness. Symptoms usually can be avoided by taking the drug with food or at bedtime and starting with low doses. For most patients, the initial recommended dosage is half a tablet (1.25 milligrams), taken at bedtime with a snack, and then the dosage is gradually increased until serum prolactin levels are normal. Thyroid hormone administration is relatively free of side effects when dosages are monitored by appropriate blood tests.

If, in addition to hormone abnormalities, disturbances of penile blood flow, nerve transmission, or psychologic conflicts are present, the response to hormone therapy will be suboptimal at best. For this reason, a careful search for coexistent neurologic, vascular, and psychologic conditions is recommended before embarking on a course of hormone therapy.

Hormones, Impotence, and the Temporal Lobe

Our understanding of the hormonal interplay necessary for normal male sexual function continues to evolve. Medical professionals used to consider the pituitary the master gland, doling out specific instructions to regulate the function of the other endocrine glands—thyroid, adrenals, and testicles. Twenty years ago it became clear that the pituitary could not discharge this important regulatory function on its own but was beholden to a higher hormonal power located in the hypothalamus. The pituitary was then more properly recognized as an intermediary existing to fulfill the hormone directives issued by the hypothalamus.

Just as we became comfortable with this concept, another

area of the brain, the temporal lobe, entered the playing field. The role of the temporal lobe in hormone secretion appears to be more meddlesome than regulatory. This is especially true when viewing the effect of temporal lobe influences on male sexual function.

Scientists studying the temporal lobe in humans were fully aware of its critical role in the reproductive and sexual function of animals. Experimental destruction of a specific portion of the temporal lobe (the amygdala) caused testicular degeneration in male rats and cats. Implants of estrogen in rabbits' amygdalae provoked hyperprolactinemia. But how do these animal experiments relate to humans?

As mentioned, some men suffer from a temporal lobe disorder called temporal lobe epilepsy (TLE). They have decreased libido and are often impotent. Some of these men have low serum testosterone levels; others have increased blood levels of prolactin.

TLE is different from other forms of epilepsy. Early symptoms are subtle and are characterized by a series of "spells." Sudden attacks of abdominal pain, dizziness, fugue states, bed-wetting, and rage as well as auditory hallucinations may be clues to the presence of a temporal lobe disorder. The coexistence of a form of epilepsy and a hormone disorder initially created a dilemma for the physician: Which condition should be treated first?

Experience provided the answer. Patients with TLE and hypogonadism are, at first, unresponsive to testosterone injections, and those with TLE and hyperprolactinema do not benefit from bromocriptine. (This distinguishes them from other hypogonadal or hyperprolactinemic men.) Antiseizure medications such as phenytoin (Dilantin) or carbamazepine (Tegretol) must be the first line of treatment. Then conventional hormone therapy is beneficial. (Frequently, the antiseizure medications not only control TLE symptoms but also allow serum hormone levels to return to normal.)

The diagnosis of TLE requires specialized testing. An unusual type of brain wave test, the sleep-deprived electroencephalogram (EEG), detects subtle disturbances in temporal lobe electrical activity. A new diagnostic probe, single photon emission computerized tomography (SPECT scan), may also help. The SPECT scan registers different colors in relation to blood flow. Areas of greatest blood flow in the brain show up with the whitest colors. Since increased blood flow is one characteristic of seizure-prone brain tissue, these areas light up on SPECT scan.

Hormone disorders are perhaps the most easily diagnosed causes of impotence, and hormone measurements should be an integral part of the early evaluation of the impotent man. Hormone abnormalities, once detected, can be treated with some dispatch and considerable success.

9

Medications, Chemicals, and Potency

Medication-induced impotence is common. In a survey of 1,180 men, medications were recognized as the single most common cause of impotence. The ingredients in many medications cause impotence by disrupting crucial sexual chemistry. In some cases, the agent deadens sex drive or libido. Other chemicals impede a man's ability to achieve erections; still others interfere with ejaculation. In most instances, once the cause-and-effect relationship between the medication and the sexual dysfunction is recognized and the offending substance is discontinued, sexual function returns to normal.

The conditions for which medicines capable of impairing male sexual function are routinely prescribed include high blood pressure, heart problems, elevated blood cholesterol levels, stomach ulcers, anxiety, and depression. These are among the most common medical problems treated today.

Physicians are often aware that the medications they prescribe can impair sexual function. They continue to write prescriptions for these medications for three important reasons:

1. The medication may be more effective than any other available drug.

2. The same medication that produces a sexual side effect in one patient may be benign in the majority of others. (Indeed, only a fraction of men taking the same medication will suffer some impairment in sexual function.)
3. Failure to treat may actually place the man at high risk for the subsequent development of impotence. This is especially true in hypertensive men. (See table 1 on pages 117–19 for a complete list of drugs and sexual side effects.)

Antihypertensive Therapy

Hypertension (high blood pressure) affects 60 million American men; 26 percent of men between the ages of eighteen and seventy-five have significant hypertension. Untreated hypertension represents a major risk factor for the development of stroke, heart attack, and heart disease.

Drugs that lower blood pressure work to overcome the overzealous internal systems responsible for the problem. That would be fine if these medications restricted their activity to lowering blood pressure. Unfortunately, chemicals in many effective blood-pressure-lowering medications create a dissonance in the neurologic and hormonal environment crucial for normal male sexual function.

Although we do not know exactly what causes blood pressure to rise, we have been able to study men with normal and high blood pressure and have learned the following.

• The amount of blood pumped out of the heart (cardiac output) is increased early on in the development of hypertension. Medications that decrease cardiac output, like the beta-blocker propranolol (Inderal), lower blood pressure.
• Blood released from the heart flows through the arterial circulation to deliver oxygen to all parts of the body. The arterial channels of hypertensive men are narrowed (constricted), creating a greater resistance so that blood pres-

sure must increase to blast its way through. Drugs that reverse arterial constriction (vasodilators), like hydralazine (Apresoline), decrease vascular resistance and allow blood pressure to fall. Other drugs, like clonidine (Catapres) and guanethidine (Ismelin), lower blood pressure by dampening the neurologic signals that make arteries constrict.

- Two powerful internally secreted chemicals, norepinephrine and angiotensin II, can, under the appropriate circumstances, cause arteries to constrict and blood pressure to increase. Drugs that nullify or at least blunt the impact of blood pressure stimulation by norepinephrine (prazosin [Minipres]) and angiotensin II (captopril [Capoten]) can lower blood pressure.

- Excessive salt (sodium overload) has long been suspected of playing a pivotal role in the development of hypertension. Desalting the body with a diuretic medication (fluid pill) has proven an effective treatment to control salt overload and help normalize blood pressure.

Today, physicians have at their disposal a wide variety of drugs capable of lowering blood pressure. Many have sexual side effects. Avoiding treatment because of fear of sexual side effects is not the answer. Untreated hypertensive men are especially vulnerable to similar sexual problems. It is only recently that the significance of this observation has been fully appreciated.

Studies of Hypertensive Men

The regularity with which antihypertensive medications affect sexual ability has prompted doctors to ponder how this comes about. Is it the fall in blood pressure, the type of medication used, or some other factor unique to men with high blood pressure that is responsible for their loss of sexual function?

Although antihypertensive medications have been available for almost fifty years, it was not until the early 1980s that several research groups decided to examine the sexual performance of untreated hypertensive men. They uncovered some unexpected information.

Hypertensive men scheduled to be enrolled in one treatment program or another were, for the first time, asked to complete questionnaires that addressed health-related issues regarding life-style, stresses, smoking and drinking habits, and prior illness. The survey also asked about any recent changes in sexual desire, difficulty obtaining or sustaining an erection, and problems ejaculating. Similar questionnaires were administered to men with normal blood pressure.

It turned out that 17 percent of hypertensive men reported difficulty achieving or sustaining an erection, compared with only 7 percent of men with normal blood pressure. Untreated hypertensive men described erectile difficulties, ejaculatory problems, and depressed libido about twice as often as other men of the same age. Thus, the framework for sexual function of hypertensive men is precarious even before treatment.

What happens to the sexual function of hypertensive men when they take medication that lowers blood pressure? The answer seems to depend on what type of medication is used and whether one or more than one antihypertensive medication is prescribed.

Physicians at the Veterans Administration have devised a Sexual Symptoms Distress Index (SSDI), which differs from other questionnaires because it does not rely solely on yes-or-no responses. Hypertensive men were asked to indicate how upset they were about a specific symptom relative to their sexual function. During the previous month, had they experienced any decreased interest in sex, problems in acquiring or maintaining an erection, or difficulty with ejaculation? Possible responses varied from "not at all" to "extremely"; scores ranged from 0 to 16. A higher number indicated greater distress.

About 40 percent of untreated hypertensive men described some dissatisfaction with sex, whereas 60 percent of men who had received some antihypertensive therapy gave a positive response to these questions.

Subsequent findings were equally enlightening. In one study men were treated first with a single antihypertensive medication—captopril (Capoten), methyldopa (Aldomet), or propranolol (Inderal). When blood pressure was not satisfactorily controlled with any of these medications alone, a second drug, the diuretic hydrochlorothiazide (HydroDIURIL), was added. To gauge sexual distress, the SSDI was administered before, during, and after therapies.

Patients receiving captopril, methyldopa, or propranolol alone had no further deterioration in sexual function. Those who were initially potent remained potent; those with already marginal SSDI scores were unchanged over the first treatment period (lasting twenty-four weeks). However, men taking methyldopa or propranolol experienced a significant deterioration of sexual function when the diuretic was added. (The diuretic had no effect on men taking captopril.) This was not entirely unexpected. Physicians already knew that methyldopa or propranolol, when administered in high doses, can impair male sexual function. Captopril does not appear to be burdened with any similar intrinsic properties. For that reason, hypertensive men treated with captopril seem to tolerate the addition of a diuretic without suffering any further sexual dysfunction.

Diuretic Medications

There are three types of diuretic medications useful in the treatment of hypertension: hydrochlorothiazide and other thiazides, furosemide (Lasix), and spironolactone (Aldactone). To date, furosemide has demonstrated no sexual side effects. However, there is a definite increase in impotence among men treated with thiazides.

Spironolactone has well-documented antiandrogen (antimale hormone) properties. Men treated with spironolactone are incapable of appreciating the full impact of their testosterone. This may explain why decreased libido is the single most common sexual side effect reported by them. Despite its side effects, spironolactone has not been stricken from the pharmacologic registry. This medication distinguishes itself from other diuretics by its ability to allow the body to flush out excess sodium while capturing potassium. All the other diuretic medications create a potassium deficiency, a condition which can cause irregular heart rhythms, constipation, muscle cramps, and—as if this were not enough—impotence.

Methyldopa

Methyldopa (Aldomet) is generally accepted as an effective antihypertensive medication, but it interferes with the function of the naturally occurring body chemical dopamine, which is important for normal nerve function and hormone release.

The body converts the drug methyldopa to a look-alike chemical called methyldopamine, which then shoulders aside the body's own dopamine. Methyldopamine is referred to as a false neurotransmitter and, like a false prophet, confuses the body by providing scrambled and inaccurate information. The result is that systems crucial for erection do not function properly. Methyldopamine also tricks the body into releasing excessive amounts of the sexually inhibiting hormone prolactin (see chapter 8). In addition, methyldopamine creates sufficient biochemical bewilderment in nerve endings to interfere with the way nerves that regulate erections communicate with one another. This then provides a favorable milieu for the development of neurogenic impotence.

The most common sexual side effects of methyldopa are decreased libido and impotence; these side effects are not universal, however. The frequency of methyldopa-induced sexual dysfunction varies from study to study, with reports ranging from as low as 3 percent to as high as 37 percent. In most series sexual side effects can be anticipated to occur in about 20 to 25 percent of methyldopa-treated hypertensive men.

Beta-Blockers

A group of medications referred to as beta-adrenergic blockers have enjoyed widespread popularity in treating high blood pressure and many heart problems. Among these medications, the beta-blocker propranolol (Inderal) has been available for the longest period, and most of our current knowledge has been derived from the experiences of hypertensive men treated with this drug.

Impotence induced by propranolol appears to be dose related. Sexual potency has been preserved in most men taking doses of up to 160 milligrams a day. When the dose is increased to 320 milligrams a day, impotence and reduced libido occur. Men with hypertension are advanced to this higher dose only if more conventional doses have not adequately controlled their blood pressure. It is not known whether it is the severity of high blood pressure alone or in combination with the increased dose of propranolol that is responsible for the sexual problems.

Metoprolol (Lopressor) is the only other beta-blocker currently acknowledged to cause sexual side effects by impairing erectile and ejaculatory function. As with propranolol, the sexual side effects of metoprolol seem dose related, with decreased libido and impotence more likely to occur at doses greater than 50 milligrams daily.

Alpha-Blockers

Guanethidine (Ismelin), prazosin (Minipres), and tetrazosin (Hytrin) disrupt the body's ability to release norepinephrine. This results in a significant fall in blood pressure, an effect that may be long lasting. The drugs also paralyze the ability of the bladder sphincter to close, preventing semen from being ejaculated from the penis. When taken for a long time, guanethidine may also interfere with the neurologic impulses required for erection, eventually leading to neurogenic impotence. Almost 100 percent of men treated with guanethidine have retrograde ejaculations and experience impotence. The drug is now used only for men whose high blood pressure is resistant to all other antihypertensives.

Prazosin and tetrazosin also have been implicated as causes of impotence and retrograde ejaculation, but less frequently.

Labetalol (Normodyne, Trandate) has both beta- and alpha-blocking properties. It, too, can cause retrograde ejaculation.

Reserpine

Reserpine is an ancient Hindu medicine originally used to treat insomnia, hyperactivity, and insanity. It was this latter property that initially attracted Western pharmacologists. Reserpine (Serpasil) was one of the first major tranquilizers introduced for the treatment of severely disturbed psychotic individuals. As psychiatrists gained familiarity with this medication, they rapidly became aware that their reserpine-treated patients had very low blood pressure and often fainted. In 1955 the pharmaceutical industry elected to capitalize on this side effect; it abandoned reserpine as an antipsychotic medication and reintroduced it as an antihypertensive drug.

A plethora of blood-pressure-lowering medicines are available today, but in the late 1950s no other antihypertensive medications existed. Thus reserpine enjoyed widespread popularity. However, it produced a number of significant and troublesome side effects, including depression, impotence, decreased libido, and an inability to ejaculate.

Reserpine interferes with the normal biochemical interactions of the neurotransmitters in the brain, which allow brain cells to communicate with one another. Reserpine-treated patients, like methyldopa-treated patients, commonly develop increased production of prolactin, a sexually inhibiting hormone. Reserpine also has a stultifying effect on the nerves that regulate erections and ejaculations. It can also lower libido. Reserpine is used rarely, only when other antihypertensive medications fail to control blood pressure.

Clonidine

Normally, neurologic impulses arising from the medulla (a portion of the brain stem) maintain blood pressure in an acceptable range. When this system overreacts, blood vessels throughout the body narrow and the force needed to propel circulating blood through these constricted arteries must increase. Clonidine (Catapres) lowers blood pressure by blunting the overactive neural signals originating in the medulla.

Clonidine is capable of exerting similar dampening effects on neurologic impulses elsewhere in the body, particularly those responsible for erection and ejaculation. The sexual side effects of clonidine appear to be both patient and dose specific. Some patients experience sexual dysfunction at any dose. Others note some sexual function impairment only at doses greater than 0.6 milligrams per day.

Calcium Channel Inhibitors

Verapamil (Calan, Isoptin), nifedipine (Procardia), and diltiazem (Cardizem) belong to a class of recently developed medications called calcium channel inhibitors. These drugs may lower blood pressure by dilating blood vessels. Isolated cases of impotence induced by calcium channel blockers have been reported, but it is too early to determine whether the group as a whole causes consistent sexual side effects.

Angiotensin-Converting Enzyme Inhibitors

One group of antihypertensive medications known as angiotensin-converting enzyme (ACE) inhibitors—captopril (Capoten) and enalapril (Vasotec)—have not caused sexual side effects to date. However, lisinopril (Zestril), a long-acting ACE inhibitor, decreases libido and causes impotence in 1 percent of treated men.

The blood-pressure-lowering effect of these ACE inhibitors is complex. They prevent the transformation of one internal chemical, angiotensin I, to another, angiotensin II. Angiotensin I has no effect on blood pressure, but angiotensin II is the most powerful blood-pressure-elevating chemical known.

Selection of an Antihypertensive Medication

What compels physicians to prescribe an antihypertensive medication with sexual side effects when they could just as easily prescribe a medication that does not have any adverse effects on male sexual function? Why are all these antihypertensive medications with sexual side effects still cluttering up pharmacists' shelves? Shouldn't they be relocated to some drugstore purgatory where they can atone for all the grief they have caused?

It is impossible to speak for all physicians, but it is likely that the following considerations enter into the ultimate decision regarding selection of a blood-pressure-lowering medicine.

Harnessing hypertension and bringing blood pressure into the normal range is the primary goal of any antihypertensive therapy. Often this can be accomplished by prescribing a single medication without any sexual side effects. However, hypertension is not always so readily managed. Nothing is gained by prescribing a medication that allows a temporary preservation of sexual function at the expense of unrestrained and uncontrolled hypertension. The risks of eventual stroke or heart attack are too great. It is in those instances, when hypertension cannot be adequately controlled by the more sexually benign medications, that a decision to add medications with potential sexual side effects must be considered. The choice is not easy. Often a satisfactory compromise can be reached so that moderating the doses of medication allows blood pressure to be controlled and sexual function retained.

Abrupt discontinuation of some of the antihypertensive medications can have dire consequences, such as striking rebound elevations in blood pressure. Patients are at risk for headache, heart symptoms, stroke (rarely), and recurrence of sexual problems.

Martin, whose father and grandfather had died of complications of hypertension, was not surprised when he learned that his blood pressure was elevated. He eagerly accepted the doctor's recommendations for an antihypertensive medication, spironolactone (Aldactone). He had no problems for three or four months, during which time he and his wife enjoyed a constant level of sexual activity. Then gradually, almost imperceptibly, he started to lose interest in sex. He no longer made sexual advances to his wife and indeed rebuffed most of her advances to him. She became agitated and suspected he was having an affair, which he vigorously denied. On reflection, they realized that the onset of his sexual apathy emerged shortly after he started to take spironolactone. He discontinued his medication, and in two or three weeks sexual desire returned. But now Martin had a new sexual problem. He could no longer acquire an erection. Blood pressure was once again elevated, requiring treatment. An alternate antihypertensive drug less likely to cause sexual side effects was substituted. As blood pressure normalized, erections and sexual intercourse resumed.

Psychiatric Medications

Most medications useful in the treatment of anxiety, depression, mania, psychotic states, and other psychiatric disorders have sexual side effects. Sexual function, however, is rarely entirely normal in psychiatric patients. Like untreated hypertensive males, men plagued by anxiety, depression, and other psychiatric disorders commonly have impaired sexual function.

Psychiatric, or psychoactive, drugs interact with the network of chemicals called neurotransmitters that are present in the brain and elsewhere in the nervous system. Neurotransmitters allow nerve cells to interact with one another. Many experts postulate that psychiatric illness reflects an ill-defined breakdown in the normal chemical communication among brain cells. This disruption favors a pattern of random, chaotic neurochemical signals that may cause depression, paranoia, psychosis, mania, or other forms of psychiatric dysfunction. Psychoactive medications are thought to be effective by virtue of their ability to redress this internal chemical turmoil and help realign neurochemical impulses so that normal communications can resume.

Psychiatric medications also interrupt the neurochemistry required for the smooth progression of the normal male sexual response cycle. Like antihypertensive medications, some psychiatric medications have a negative effect on libido and/or impair the capability to have erections. But the most consistently reported sexual side effect is delayed ejaculation or a complete inability to ejaculate.

Antidepressant Medications

Decreased libido and impotence are common in men suffering from depression. Sexual function usually returns to normal when the depression lifts with treatment. Antidepressant medications fall into three general classes of drugs: tricyclic antidepressants (Imipramine, Desipramine, Amitriptyline, Nortriptyline), monoamine oxidase (MAO) inhibitors (Phenelzine, Isocarboxacid, Tranylcypromine), and atypical antidepressants (Trazodone). Sexual side effects are common with all these drugs. Even the newest antidepressant, fluoxetine (Prozac), has been recognized to inhibit orgasm in 8 percent of cases.

The scenario sounds ominously familiar, something like an instant replay of the hypertension-antihypertensive therapy conundrum. There are indeed similarities, but there are also notable differences.

- Although it is true that compromised sexual function is one of the hallmarks of depression, it is equally apparent that for the sexually dysfunctional man resurrection of sexual prowess occurs only when his depression is alleviated. Impotent hypertensive men often experience, but cannot depend on, a similar improvement in sexual function when their blood pressure is normalized.

- The trend in tracking sexual function of hypertensive men before, during, and after therapy has not yet established a strong foothold in psychiatric literature. As a result, most of our information regarding the sexual side effects of psychiatric drugs has been derived from either anecdotal individual case reports or sidebars to scientific papers describing both the effectiveness and adverse effects of new antidepressant medications.
- The scale of studies exploring antidepressant-induced sexual side effects is not comparable. The experiences of thousands of hypertensive men now provide the foundation for our knowledge of the sexual side effects of antihypertensive medications. The largest single report of psychoactive drug-induced impairment in sexual function is based on interviews of fifty-seven men who were already receiving the antipsychotic medication thioridazine (Mellaril) at the time of the interview. Impaired ejaculation was reported by twenty-eight of the men (49 percent).
- Paradoxically, the most common sexual side effect of psychoactive drugs has proven to be a boon to some men with other specific sexual dysfunctions. We know that antidepressant and antipsychotic medications commonly cause delayed or retarded ejaculation. This side effect is a godsend for men suffering from premature ejaculation. Unfortunately, none of the sexual side effects of antihypertensive medications can be similarly adapted to improve the lot of other sexually dysfunctional men.
- Priapism is one sexual side effect attributed to psychiatric medications not shared by the antihypertensives. This painful persistent erection has been recognized with increasing frequency in men who take antidepressant medications. Several tricyclic and MAO inhibitor antidepressants have been reported to cause priapism on rare occasions. Trazodone (Desyrel), an atypical antidepressant, also has been implicated as causing priapism.

Antipsychotic Medications

Schizophrenia and other major emotional disorders can be treated by three groups of medications referred to as antipsychotic drugs: phenothiazines, thioxanthenes, and butyrophenones. Medications from each group have been incriminated as causes of sexual dysfunction, but exact knowledge of the patient's normal sexual function *prior* to initiation of the drug is often lacking. Thus, the best evidence comes from the occasional patient who reports problems with sexual function when he starts treatment with a different antipsychotic medication. Inhibition of ejaculation is a common sexual side effect associated with thioridazine (Mellaril), as noted, and other phenothiazine medications as well. In a few patients, thioridazine also inhibited libido and erections.

The grandfather of all phenothiazine medications, chlorpromazine (Thorazine), is also known to cause inhibited ejaculation. Chlorpromazine has been evaluated in a carefully controlled study that found it does not interfere with erections or libido.

Fluphenazine (Prolixin) has been saddled with the designation of a libido-inhibiting medication as a result of a report that described the effectiveness of fluphenazine in inhibiting the desire of men convicted of sexual crimes. A large dose of fluphenazine given by injection did produce some reduction in their libido.

Nevertheless, inhibited ejaculation remains the single most common side effect of the mainstream antipsychotic psychiatric medications.

Lithium

Lithium, usually in the form of lithium carbonate (Lithobid, Eskalith), is used to treat patients with mania. Mania is a condition of hyperactivity and disordered thinking that may occur spontaneously, as an independent illness, but more often occurs in conjunction with depression. People affected with the dual illnesses of depression and mania are said to have a "bipolar disorder." Antidepressant therapy is appropriate when they are in the depressed phase of their illness, but when the manic phase supervenes, treatment with lithium is warranted.

Some patients in a manic phase complain that lithium induces sexual side effects, but the data supporting this conclusion are shaky at best. When patients are manic, they have an exaggerated sense of their own sexual prowess. Therefore, it is impossible to obtain accurate baseline information regarding the sexual function of actively manic patients unless their partners can provide corroborating evidence. As the mania and hyperactivity come under control, the patient's thinking becomes more properly attuned to reality.

It is difficult to know whether the impotence reported by some patients in the course of lithium therapy is actually caused by the medication. In the most widely quoted study, two of ten lithium-treated patients developed impotence. Potency returned in both, one who stopped and another who continued lithium treatment. For this reason, it remains unclear whether lithium alone has any negative effect on male sexual function.

Minor Tranquilizers

Millions of minor tranquilizers are taken every day to relieve anxiety, relax muscle tension, and help people fall asleep. Included are chlordiazepoxide (Librium), diazepam (Valium), lorazepam (Ativan), alprazolam (Xanax), and clorazepate (Tranxene). It is unclear whether these medications have any effect on male sexual function.

Antiulcer Medications

Physicians often prescribe cimetidine (Tagamet) for gastritis and ulcers because it inhibits acid production by the stomach. Cimetidine also inhibits testosterone production, and men treated with it often complain of impotence. When cimetidine therapy is stopped, the stimulus for testosterone secretion resumes and potency is restored.

Ranitidine (Zantac) and famotidine (Pepcid) are similar to cimetidine. Both drugs are equally effective in decreasing production of stomach acid, but neither appears to cause sexual side effects.

Cholesterol-Lowering Medications

Clofibrate (Atromid-S) lowers serum cholesterol levels. Unfortunately, the same properties that allow it to inhibit cholesterol production also interfere with the testicle's ability to manufacture testosterone. As expected, men treated with clofibrate often complain of diminished libido and impotence.

None of the other cholesterol-lowering drugs appears to interfere with sexual function.

Our current knowledge of the neurologic, vascular, and hormonal interplay necessary for normal male sexual function, though imperfect, is still sufficiently advanced to allow us to understand how prescription drugs and other ingested chemicals can disrupt all or part of the sexual response cycle and cause impotence and infertility.

The physical systems necessary for potency and fertility are remarkably resilient but not infinitely elastic. Some prescription drugs used to treat high blood pressure and emotional disorders have sexual side effects; others do not. Nevertheless, control of the blood pressure and emotional disorder is of paramount importance to health. If the physician can achieve this goal without compromising sexual function, he or she will do so. But this is not always possible. Occasionally, once inroads in the control of blood pressure or emotional disorders have been achieved by a medication with sexual side effects, a physician can adjust the dosage to sustain the therapeutic benefit; doses of the sexually noxious drug are gradually discontinued, and a second drug without sexual side effects is introduced. This tricky business requires close collaboration between doctor and patient.

In addition to the pills supplied by physicians to treat medical conditions, surgical procedures (see chapter 10) performed to alleviate major, sometimes life-threatening illnesses can, as an unintended effect, create impotence. In situations where a physician, either by prescribing a medication or by performing surgery, causes an unanticipated side effect, the resultant problem is said to be "iatrogenic" (from *iatros*, Greek for "physician").

However, physicians are not the sole purveyors of impotence-causing chemicals.

Self-Administered Substances That Affect Potency

Cigarettes

Heavy cigarette smoking damages the large arteries supplying blood to all areas of the pelvis and limits the amount of blood available for erections. In addition, and perhaps more important, cigarette smoking damages the tiny blood vessels in the penis that must enlarge to accept the substantial onrush of blood expected during the course of normal erection.

Autopsy studies of heavy smokers show that the small arterioles in the penis are universally narrowed, scarred, and no longer retain the elasticity needed to expand. In contrast, the small penile blood vessels of nonsmokers are normal. This is true for both young and old men alike.

It is no longer necessary to rely solely on anatomic specimens to demonstrate the negative impact of cigarettes on male sexual function. The same information can be obtained by examining the smoking habits of men enrolled in impotence clinics. In two separate surveys, cigarette smoking among impotent men was two times higher than in the normal male population. Over 58 percent of impotent men were active smokers, and 81 percent admitted to heavy cigarette use in the past.

The rate of blood flow into the penis can be measured and calculated as a penile brachial index (PBI) (see chapter 7). Impotent men who are heavy smokers have a clearly subnormal PBI, indicating that blood flow is inadequate for normal erections.

It is believed that when men stop smoking, penile blood vessels can reconstitute themselves to allow for normal blood flow and restoration of erectile capability. As with any other type of cigarette-induced vascular disease, the critical factor allowing recovery seems to be the number of cigarettes smoked and the duration of the smoking habit.

It is not yet clear how much cigarette smoking a man can tolerate without compromising his sexual function. In dogs, the inhaled smoke from only two cigarettes impairs canine erectile function. In the human, casual smoking may not have a deleterious effect. However, irreparable damage to the penile blood vessels and impaired erectile capability appear to be inevitable for men who smoke packs or fractions of packs a day for several decades.

Alcohol

The negative effect of alcohol consumption on sexual function has been known for many years. Shakespeare was well aware of the initially disinhibiting but ultimately intrusive role of alcohol. In *Macbeth,* the porter says, "It [drink] provokes the desire, but it takes away the performance."

It is possible that moderate alcohol consumption provides some tranquilizing benefit to alleviate sexual anxieties. However, the adverse effects of excessive alcohol consumption on sexual performance have been well documented and commonly experienced. Many fully potent men can recall an episode of alcohol-induced impotence. This is primarily due to the soporific effect of alcohol. Inebriated or only slightly tipsy men planning to have sex find that there is a point when the sedative effects of alcohol overcome its disinhibiting effects. In such cases libido is squelched in favor of a good night's sleep.

Several critical functions necessary for normal male sexual activity are temporarily or irreparably impaired by excessive alcohol consumption. Alcohol inhibits the ability of the testicle to produce testosterone, the major hormone responsible for sex drive or libido. Alcoholic men with low serum testosterone levels have little or no interest in sex.

Alcohol-induced liver damage causes a shift in testosterone metabolism so that this vital male hormone is shunted away from the path that leads to the creation of the even more potent male hormone dihydrotestosterone (DHT) and into a direction that favors the increased production of a female hormone, an estrogen called estradiol (E_2). Inappropriate high serum estrogen levels cause alcoholic men to have enlarged breasts and a characteristic flushing of the face and palms.

The reproductive function of the testicle is also impaired by heavy drinking. Infertility is a common result.

Alcohol damages the nerves that allow erection and ejaculation to occur. Many alcoholics are unable to produce semen by masturbation because they can no longer ejaculate forward. The nerve damage caused by alcohol results in retrograde ejaculation.

Many of these changes are reversible with abstinence. Recovery of potency and fertility is most likely in those men whose drinking has not damaged the liver or the nerves that allow erections or ejaculation to take place.

A precise itemization of the total amount of alcohol a man must consume to qualify as a heavy drinker or an alcoholic is not readily available. Most men would like to believe that an alcoholic is someone who drinks more than they do. This is an unfortunate delusion. However, it is still not known exactly how much a man can drink with impunity, or at what point his cumulative alcohol consumption is sufficient to usher him across his own sexual and reproductive Rubicon.

Marijuana

Tetrahycacannabinol (THC), the active ingredient in marijuana, is thought to have a positive effect on male sexual function by increasing sensate focus. Substantial evidence has now accumulated to indicate that chronic THC use has an adverse effect on both male sexual function and fertility. An enlargement of the male breast (gynecomastia) and a progressive decrease in serum testosterone levels have been noted in chronic marijuana users. In animals, THC use has a negative effect on sexual interest and performance and has a curiously devastating impact on the fertility of male offspring.

Mice exposed to THC in doses equivalent to three marijuana cigarettes daily have high miscarriage rates, and their offspring have a fourfold increase in chromosomal abnormalities. A trend of progressive decrease in fertility extends through the first and second generation of male mice whose parents have been exposed to marijuana. Translation of this mouse research into human terms should be available shortly as the first and second generations of male children born to parents of the Woodstock generation reach reproductive age.

Opiate Drugs

Morphine, heroin, and methadone fall into a class of drugs known as opiates. They have a profound negative effect on the hormonal regulation of male sexual function. All serve to depress the normal pattern of secretion of the hypothalamic hormones that trigger the release of LH and ultimately testosterone. Low testosterone production, decreased libido, and impotence are all common among chronic heroin, morphine, and methadone addicts.

Cocaine

Cocaine enjoys a reputation as an aphrodisiac. However, substantial evidence is accumulating to indicate that chronic cocaine use, alone or in combination with alcohol, ultimately causes sexual dysfunction. Cocaine alone stimulates secretion of the sexually inhibiting hormone prolactin. Cocaine also causes spasms in arteries; blood flow to the penis cannot be sustained if arterial spasms persist. Studies in detoxification centers have demonstrated that partner sex, masturbation, and orgasm frequency decline with chronic cocaine use. Sexual function can return to normal after cocaine detoxification and abstinence. A drug-free interval of nine months to one year is required for restoration of libido and potency.

**Table 1. Sexual Side Effects of
Common Prescription Medications**

GENERIC NAME	BRAND NAME	SEXUAL SIDE EFFECTS
Antihypertensive Medications		
Diuretics		
Spironolactone	Aldactone	Decreased libido, breast swelling, impotence
Thiazides	Diuril, HydroDIURIL, Naturetin, Naqua, many others	Impotence
Furosemide	Lasix	None
Centrally Acting		
Methyldopa	Aldomet	Decreased libido, impotence
Clonidine	Catapres	Impotence
Reserpine	Serpasil, Raudixin, Ser-Ap-Es	Decreased libido, impotence, depression
Alpha-Adrenergic Blockers		
Prazosin	Minipres	"Dry" (retrograde) ejaculation
Terazosin	Hytrin	"Dry" (retrograde) ejaculation
Beta-Adrenergic Blockers		
Propanolol	Inderal	Impotence, decreased libido
Metoprolol	Lopressor	Impotence, decreased libido
Combined Alpha- and Beta-Adrenergic Blockers		
Labetalol	Normodyne, Trandate	Inhibited ejaculation
Nonadrenergic Vasodilators		
Hydralazine	Apresoline	None
Sympathetic Nerve Blockers		
Guanethidine	Ismelin	Impotence, "dry" (retrograde) ejaculation
Angiotensin-Converting Enzyme (ACE) Inhibitors		
Captopril	Capoten	None
Enalapril	Vasotec	None
Lisinopril	Zestril	Impotence in a small percentage (1 percent) of cases

Table 1. (*continued*)

GENERIC NAME	BRAND NAME	SEXUAL SIDE EFFECTS
Psychiatric Medications		
Antidepressants		
Tricyclics		
Amitriptyline	Elavil	Inhibited ejaculation, impotence
Amoxapine	Ascendin	Decreased libido, impotence
Desipramine	Norpramin	Inhibited ejaculation
Doxepin	Sinequan	Inhibited ejaculation, impotence
Imipramine	Tofranil	Inhibited ejaculation, impotence
Maprotriline	Ludiomil	Inhibited ejaculation
Nortriptyline	Aventyl, Pamelor	Inhibited ejaculation
Protriptyline	Vivactil	Inhibited ejaculation, impotence
Atypical		
Trazodone	Desyrel	Priapism
Monoamine Oxidase (MAO) Inhibitors		
Isocarboxazid	Marplan	Inhibited ejaculation
Phenelzine	Nardil	Inhibited ejaculation, decreased libido
Tranylcypromine	Parnate	Inhibited ejaculation
Antipsychotic Medications		
Phenothiazine Group		
Thioridazine	Mellaril	Inhibited ejaculation, priapism, decreased libido
Chlorpromazine	Thorazine	Inhibited ejaculation
Mesoridazine	Serentil	Inhibited ejaculation, decreased libido
Fluphenazine	Prolixin	Inhibited ejaculation, decreased libido
Serotonin Reuptake Inhibitors		
Fluoxetine	Prozac	Anorgasmia (8 percent)
Perphenazine	Trilafon	Inhibited ejaculation
Trifluoperazine	Stelazine	Inhibited ejaculation
Thioxanthene Group		
Chlorprothixene	Taractan	Inhibited ejaculation
Thiothixene	Navane	Inhibited ejaculation, impotence
Butyrophenone		
Haloperidol	Haldol	Inhibited ejaculation
Antimania Medication		
Lithium carbonate	Eskalith, Lithobid	Possible impotence
Antiulcer Medications		
Cimetidine	Tagamet	Decreased libido, impotence, gynecomastia
Ranitidine	Zantac	None
Famotidine	Pepcid	None

Table 1. (*continued*)

GENERIC NAME	BRAND NAME	SEXUAL SIDE EFFECTS
Cholesterol-Lowering Medications		
Clofibrate	Atromid-S	Impotence
Cholestyramine	Questran	None
Colestipol	Colestid	None
Gemfibrozil	Lopid	None
Probucol	Lorelco	None
Lovastatin	Mevacor	None

10

Prostate Surgery
and Other Medical Problems

The prostate gland rests in the lower abdomen nestled between the bladder and the rectum (see figure 8). Fluid secretions from the prostate mix with sperm released from the testicles and contribute to semen. Additional fluid is provided by the seminal vesicles, smaller glands huddled near the prostate.

Most men are unaware of the presence of their prostate until it becomes inflamed, infected, or enlarged. Inflammation of the prostate (prostatitis) often causes rectal pain or pain on urination. Prostatitis is a concern for young sexually active men because it is often, but not invariably, the result of a venereal or sexually transmitted disease. Extremely painful ejaculation is a common symptom. Prostatitis can be satisfactorily controlled by antibiotics or other treatments.

Benign Prostatic Hypertrophy

Enlargement of the prostate gland occurs frequently in middle-age and older men. The more common problem is benign

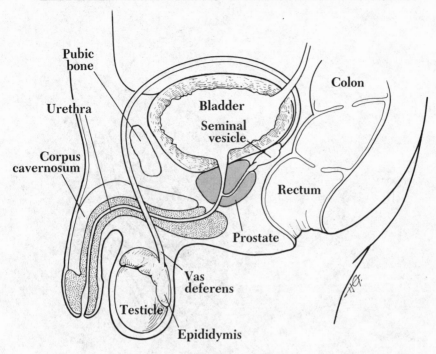

Figure 8.   Normal anatomy of prostate, bladder, and urethra in young man.

prostatic hypertrophy (BPH), a progressive increase in the size of the gland. Surgical treatment of BPH has been successful, but sexual side effects, including retrograde (or backward) ejaculation and impotence, occur with some regularity.

The proximity of the prostate to the lower end of the bladder, specifically the area where the bladder joins the urethra, is responsible for the vast majority of symptoms of an enlarged prostate. The progressive growth of the prostate creates a bulge, something like a knuckle, at the critical junction between the bladder and the urethra. Urine is, in a sense, dammed up inside the bladder (see figure 9). When this occurs, the patterns of urination change. Men urinate frequently but do not completely empty their bladder; they may be aware of some dribbling of urine out of their penis after they thought that they had finished voiding. They may also wake up frequently during the night to urinate.

The symptoms are all caused by the large prostate now re-

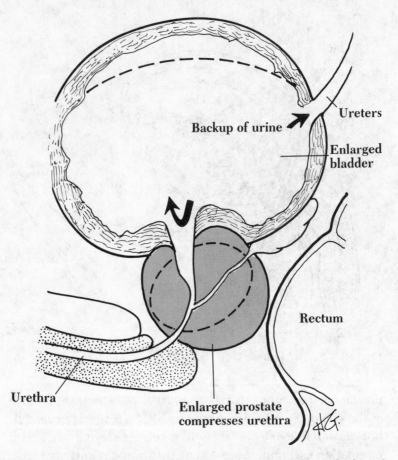

Figure 9.   Prostate enlargement compresses urethra resulting in backup of urine into the bladder.

stricting urine flow from the bladder. The problem can be corrected only by reestablishing the channel for freer urine flow. An operation called a transurethral prostatectomy (TURP) is performed by inserting a probe into the urethra to allow the urologist to visualize the area of obstruction. The doctor then shaves away prostatic tissue to reopen communication between bladder and urethra.

Men who have had a TURP experience no decrease in sexual desire and retain the ability to have erections, engage in sexual intercourse, and ejaculate. Unfortunately, the surgical procedure may cause damage to the internal bladder sphincter, the valve responsible for forward ejaculation of semen. A damaged bladder sphincter cannot close prior to ejaculation, resulting in retrograde ejaculation of semen into the bladder.

Retrograde ejaculation is clearly a major issue for men who want to produce their own offspring. Fortunately, BPH tends to affect older men. Although it is occasionally possible to retrieve semen that has been ejaculated backward into the bladder and use it for insemination, the procedure is onerous and time consuming, with only a limited success rate.

Prostate Cancer

Prostatic enlargement is not always benign. Sometimes the prostate undergoes a malignant transformation to prostate cancer. Occasionally the cancer remains contained within the confines of the prostate, and limited local surgery suffices. But when prostate cancer spreads, extensive and aggressive surgery is necessary. In the past, men who had such surgery invariably became impotent. This no longer needs to be the result.

Adjacent to the prostate are vital collections of blood vessels and nerves critical for erection. In the early 1980s, Dr. Patrick Walsh of Johns Hopkins Medical School focused his energies on these neurovascular bundles. He found that they are intimately involved in the transmission of vital signals to the spongy structures in the penis that must become engorged with blood for a fully rigid erection. If the neurovascular bodies were removed during surgery, erections would not occur.

When Dr. Walsh and his colleagues operated on patients with spreading prostatic cancer, they did so by first identifying, and then sparing, the neurovascular bundles. Their patients remained potent. It turns out that there are two neurovascular bundles, one on either side of the prostate. If both bundles are removed in an effort to rid the lower abdomen of all spreading prostate cancer during prostate surgery, men become impotent. However, if one bundle can be salvaged, potency is preserved.

Treatment for More Advanced Prostatic Cancer

Prostate tissue grows in response to stimulation from androgens, particularly the testicular hormone testosterone. Eliminate testosterone production, and the spread of prostatic cancer slows. One way to curtail testosterone production abruptly is to remove both testicles. Unfortunately, excluding testosterone from the circulation also eradicates sexual desire. There is now another way to nullify the role of testosterone without resorting to surgical castration.

As noted, the hypothalamic-pituitary-testicular system works only when it pulses. Bursts from the hypothalamus of gonadotropin releasing hormone (GnRH) act on the pituitary to trigger the release of other hormones, which in turn stimulates testosterone and sperm production. Medications are now available that cripple the pulsatile nature of this system. Drugs that are structurally similar to GnRH, for example leuprolide (Lupron), are effective in controlling prostatic cancer because they cause serum testosterone production to cease. But this treatment, too, eliminates sexual desire and stymies potency.

Other Cancer Treatments

Malignant tumors of the prostate are not the only cancers that spread to and establish a foothold in the pelvis. Cancers of the bowel, bladder, testicle, and lymphatic system often extend beyond their original boundaries as well. The spreading cancer can strangle and compromise the function of the neurovascular bundles vital for erection.

Two treatments commonly used to control these cancers— X-ray (radiation) therapy and chemotherapy—also interfere with sexual and reproductive function.

Focused radiation therapy can slow the spread of cancer in the pelvis but cannot avoid affecting the adjacent nerves and blood vessels necessary for erection. Impotence is a common result.

Chemotherapy, administered orally or intravenously, has a more selective effect. Chemotherapeutic drugs routinely cause irreparable damage to the sperm-producing units of the testicle but do not affect the testicle's ability to manufacture and release testosterone. The result is that men become infertile but retain their sexual desire and potency (see chapter 15).

11

Psychologic Factors
Affecting Potency
and Ejaculation

Our current understanding of the male sexual response cycle is based in large part on the contributions of psychiatrists, psychologists, and behavioral scientists. Until recently only they had the opportunity to delve into issues relevant to male sexual function. Others did not challenge the mental health profession's exclusive dominion over sexual matters. Sex was discussed in psychiatry and psychology textbooks only.

As a result, medical textbooks published before 1980 were not inclined to devote much attention to the subject of impotence because at that time it was commonly believed that 90 percent or more of impotence was psychologic in origin. This limited perspective has been reconsidered. Current medical textbooks discuss impotence extensively and thoroughly. Today, physicians recognize that in addition to psychologic problems, physical or organic (vascular, neurologic, or hormonal) abnormalities can disrupt the male sexual response cycle.

Whereas men with organic types of impotence have physical conditions that require correction, men with so-called psychogenic impotence are physically capable of sex but are blocked by some emotional discord. Psychogenic impotence is a generic diagnosis encompassing a constellation of problems including performance anxiety, lack of sensate focus, recent or deeply rooted emotional conflicts, and depression. Anxiety and other emotional factors may impede sexual satisfaction by causing premature or delayed ejaculation. Effective treatment is available once a correct diagnosis is made.

Symptoms and Diagnosis

Psychologic factors must be considered instrumental in a man's impotence if he:

- Has normal erections in the morning, evening, during masturbation, with an alternate sexual partner, after viewing erotic films, or any other time but is incapable of acquiring an erection when he attempts to make love with his primary partner.
- Has experienced a *sudden* loss of potency in the absence of direct injury to the spine or penis.
- Is embroiled in a fractious relationship with his partner.
- Feels under undue stress.
- Finds sexual intercourse an anxiety-provoking experience.
- Describes symptoms or shows signs compatible with a diagnosis of depression.

It is not always obvious when emotional problems are causing sexual difficulties. Being impotent is in itself a depressing and anxiety-provoking experience. All impotent men, when first evaluated, appear anxious and, if not overtly depressed, despondent about their loss of sexual function. This is true even for those men whose impotence is caused by neurologic, vascular, or hormonal abnormalities. In their case, any psychological problems are a *reaction to* and not a *cause of* their impotence.

Sometimes psychogenic impotence is the diagnosis by default. After normal nocturnal penile tumescence, penile blood flow, and hormone tests have exonerated neurologic, vascular, or hormonal systems, psychogenic impotence emerges as the only remaining fall-back diagnosis. On other occasions, the recognition of organic or psychologic causes of impotence may be solely a reflection of the type of doctor who evaluates the man: The mind-set of the examining physician exerts a powerful influence on the ultimate diagnosis. Urologists, internists, and endocrinologists are more likely to look for and find organic, rather than psychologic, causes of impotence. Psychiatrists are more attuned to recognition of subtle psychologic problems.

Evaluation and Treatment

A detailed medical history is the first step in understanding the nature of the psychologic conflict responsible for the current sexual problem (see chapter 5).

A battery of pencil-and-paper tests, in the form of self- or therapist-administered questionnaires, are also available to help establish a psychologic profile of men with sexual problems. The Multiaxial Descriptive System for Sexual Dysfunction Manual (MADSSDM) provides a format for the precise classification of sexual problems. Questions are designed to illuminate specific details of a man's current and prior sexual activity, desires, fetishes, and concerns. More elaborate probes have been devised to assess his level of sexual knowledge and misconceptions. Still others explore the nature of the man's sexual fantasies and experiences and ask him to describe his level of satisfaction with his current and prior sexual partners.

These questionnaires are valuable research tools, but do not by themselves confirm a diagnosis of psychogenic impotence. Information provided by these questionnaires can only establish the baseline level of sexual dysfunction. During and after therapy the questionnaires can be readministered to determine whether medication, psychotherapy, or sex therapy was effective.

A wide variety of services are now offered impotent men with psychologic problems. Psychiatrists, psychologists, sex therapists, and specially trained counselors can all provide help; discussion between therapist and patient (or "talk therapy") is the primary form of treatment for psychologic problems. Sex therapists can furnish the patient with additional sexual information and education. The patient may need medications, either mild tranquilizers or more powerful antidepressants. In such cases, the services of a psychiatrist are necessary.

At the outset, it must be determined whether the dysfunction is primary or secondary.

Primary Impotence

Men with primary impotence have never experienced normal psychosexual maturation, nor have they ever successfully masturbated or engaged in a satisfactory sexual relationship. For many years primary impotence was believed to be a relatively rare problem. In his *Sexual Behavior in the Human Male,* Dr. Alfred Kinsey reported that less than 0.4 percent of men under the age of twenty-five had primary impotence. It is possible that this figure underestimated the prevalence of this disorder.

A recent reawakening of interest in the subject of male sexual problems and the availability of treatment has unearthed a cache of men with primary impotence. In one recent study of 573 consecutive men seen at an impotence clinic in a German military hospital, 67 (11.7 percent) had primary erectile dysfunction. All 67 men gave a history of a total absence of fully sustained erections since early childhood or puberty. Surprisingly, physical abnormalities were detected in 57 (85 percent) of them. Only 15 percent had purely psychogenic impotence. However, all of them, even those with organic causes of their impotence, also had significant psychologic difficulties, possibly as a secondary reaction to their lifelong inability to function sexually. The results of the German study have not yet been confirmed elsewhere. In most physicians' experience, psychologic problems dominate in men with primary impotence.

Effective treatment of men with primary impotence is extraordinarily difficult and often fails. Men with primary impotence who have vascular or neurologic problems must first have the physical defect corrected. Vascular surgery is possible in some cases to reestablish blood flow to the genitalia. Disrupted neurologic connections are less amenable to correction. Circuitous methods to bypass the nerve damage either by inserting a penile prosthesis or by using intrapenile injections to stimulate erections can be considered. Either technique allows the man to experience erections.

Treatment of physical problems is a start, but it does not provide a fully satisfactory or comprehensive treatment. Psychotherapy is necessary to help the man arrive at some understanding of the physical and emotional factors that contributed to his long-term inability to function sexually. With insight gained from therapy, he should be able to enjoy some sexual satisfaction.

Ralph was thirty-seven years old when he was seen in consultation, ostensibly for evaluation of infertility. The reason for the barren marriage surfaced when Ralph indicated that he and his wife had never had sexual intercourse. Further probing revealed an unfathomable depth of sexual naivete.

Ralph had grown up in a strictly religious household and was made to feel ashamed of the erections he had as an adolescent. He did not know what masturbation meant. His teenage years at an all-boys military school provided no enlightenment, for he was shy and reclusive. When asked if he knew how men and women had babies, he responded, "I just get on top and then do it."

Studies indicated that Ralph was able to have erections and had a normal complement of hormones. An enormous chunk of life, critical for normal psychosexual development, was either not developed or repressed. Ralph was referred to a group of psychologists to see if they could resurrect fragments of his lost adolescence, a daunting task even for the most confident therapist.

This condition, primary impotence, though startling and dramatic, is the exception and not the rule.

Secondary Impotence

The majority of sexually dysfunctional men have secondary impotence. At one time they engaged in sexual activity and were able to acquire and sustain an erection satisfactory for masturbation or intercourse. Then something happened to stifle their natural sexual urges, inhibit erectile capabilities, or meddle with the ejaculatory process.

Details of the vascular anatomy, neurologic connections, and patterns of hormone secretion required for normal male sexual function have already been spelled out. With specific testing we can recognize abnormalities in blood flow to the penis, neurologic impulses, and hormone disorders. The psychological prerequisites are somewhat more difficult to define. Dr. Steven Levine, a psychiatrist at Case Western Reserve University in Cleveland, has identified the psychological underpinnings for a satisfactory sexual life as "a willingness to make love, capacity to relax, and the ability to concentrate on sensation." Yet how can we determine whether somebody's "willingness to make love" is impaired? How do we gauge his "capacity to relax" or his "ability to concentrate on sensation"? These emotional factors cannot be measured with any precision. All we can do is provide some sense of their impact on sexual function by way of illustration, using performance anxiety as one prototype of psychogenic impotence.

Performance Anxiety

Performance anxiety is one of the most common sexual problems. A man, fully potent for most of his life, suddenly experiences a sexual failure. He is surprised to find that while having sex he can neither achieve nor sustain an erection satisfactory to complete the sexual act.

Men respond to this problem in different ways. Some assume that the failure was a temporary nuisance that will resolve itself spontaneously. They do not dwell on one isolated incident and indeed have no difficulty having an erection the next time they attempt sexual intercourse.

Other men become preoccupied with their ability to achieve an erection. The sexual act shifts from a sensual, erotic experience to a worrisome encounter. The man becomes obsessed with the transition of his penis from a limp to an erect state. Each time he attempts intercourse he wonders whether he will be able to have an erection, and if so, for how long. These concerns are difficult to extinguish. The man becomes so consumed with them that all other components of the sexual act lose importance. He is, in a sense, staring at his penis like a spectator waiting to see if the erection will occur and praying that once it does occur it will not fade.

The term *spectatoring* has been coined to describe this phenomenon. The focus on the penis consumes the man to the exclusion of all other sexual thoughts. The "willingness to make love" has been replaced by an "anxiety over the ability to make love." The cycle is vicious. The more he concentrates on his penis to see if it will become erect, the more he is destined to fail. A series of failures begets more anxiety, which in turn guarantees further failure.

What commonly follows is a cascade of events that makes things worse. First he withdraws, avoiding routine intimate and even conventional physical contact, such as hugging and kissing. His anxiety about his inability to perform becomes intense. Soon he ceases all sensual contact and feels broken and diminished by his impotence.

One pragmatic treatment approach accepts a man's sexual dysfunction and impotence as a fact and does not inquire into the source of the problem. Treatments are designed to help him restore his willingness to make love, capacity to relax, and ability to concentrate on sensation. These are the sensate focus exercises popularized by Masters and Johnson.

Sensate Focus Exercises

Twenty years after their landmark book, *Human Sexual Inadequacy*, William Masters and Virginia Johnson's treatment programs are still used. Some have quibbled with certain aspects of their program, but the fundamental principles remain sound.

Lack of sensate focus was considered by Masters and Johnson to be the most common, potentially remediable, sexual problem experienced by men. Men can often be distracted during sex by unrelated, troublesome thoughts. These nettlesome concerns inhibit a man's ability to concentrate on sensation. As a result, a man experiencing lack of sensate focus does not achieve an erection during foreplay. Even if an erection sufficient for penetration does occur, it cannot be maintained while his mind is preoccupied.

The original Masters and Johnson technique was developed for couples who were willing to devote two weeks to an intensive daily sexual therapy program. Male and female cotherapists were a critical component of the treatment. Today, similar programs continue the dual-therapist approach; other equally successful programs are directed by a single therapist and usually extend over several weeks to months. Common to all programs is a set of ground rules:

1. Couples must agree to establish a moratorium on sexual intercourse during the treatment period. They are not permitted even to attempt intercourse until directed to do so by the therapist.
2. They must have no extramarital affairs during the course of therapy.
3. The use of alcohol, mood-altering drugs, or nonprescription medications must stop.
4. Both partners must agree to set apart a specific time of the day to do individual homework assignments.
5. The couple must start with a clean slate, setting aside any disagreements or grievances.
6. They must be explicit in telling each other what does and does not stimulate them.

Although it is true that Masters and Johnson are properly credited with popularizing sensate focus programs today, similar exercises were first proposed more than two hundred years ago. In 1788 the English surgeon Dr. John Hunter first prescribed "six amatory experiences without coital connexion." Even in the eighteenth century physicians recognized the need to reestablish a sense of erotic arousal with "amatory exercises" in a setting that temporarily prohibited sexual intercourse "without coital connexion."

Today the same principles have been resurrected. The original sensate focus exercises have been modified and adapted primarily to accommodate the busy schedule of working men and women. The goal is unchanged. The sensate focus exercises seek to reawaken sexual desire and allow couples to become comfortable and relaxed during the sexual experience.

The treatment begins with a reexamination and discussion of female and male sensual anatomy. Men and women are encouraged to identify those forms of stimulation that excite and those that diminish their sexual desire. Discovering maneuvers that turn on and turn off sexual interest is most important at this early phase. This information is especially useful for couples who are no longer aroused by the pattern of lovemaking that they had once found exciting.

It is also critical that the man be absolved of any anxiety he may harbor about achieving erections. The physiology of erections and their *involuntary* regulation by neurologic, vascular, and hormonal influences are stressed. At this time the man is encouraged to dispel all notions that he should be able to have an "erection on demand." Rather, he is encouraged to concentrate on the sensations that arouse him and communicate about them to the woman. She, in turn, must help him appreciate what excites her.

The actual sequence of sensate focus maneuvers is programmed as different levels of exercises performed over several days or weeks. During this time, attempts at intercourse are forbidden. The goal of the exercises is to reawaken sexual desire and allow couples to become comfortable and relaxed during sex.

Sensate Focus Exercises

Step 1. Lie together naked, hold each other, breathe together, but do not touch sexually sensitive areas.

Step 2. Explore all parts of the body manually or orally but exclude the breasts and genitals. The partners are encouraged to take turns so that both can find ways to relax and arouse each other.

Step 3. Breast caressing. Manual or oral stimulation of the breast is allowed at this time.

Step 4. The woman is encouraged to caress the man's penis and scrotum. The goal is not to achieve erection or orgasm but to create an atmosphere for a pleasurable experience.

Step 5. Manual caressing of the genitals to bring both partners to orgasm. During this phase concern is raised about premature ejaculation. The woman is instructed in the "squeeze" or "start-stop" exercises to delay the moment of ejaculation.

Step 6. Intercourse is allowed, but the goal is simply vaginal penetration. Only a minimum amount of thrusting is permitted. To make matters easier for the man, he is advised to lie on his back with the woman on top.

Step 7. An extension of step six. Intercourse with prolonged thrusting to orgasm. Again the women is on top.

Step 8. Allows intercourse with the man on top.

Therapists usually instruct patients to proceed very slowly through the sensate focus sequence and encourage repetition of each step for several nights before moving on to the next. If problems surface, the couple is encouraged to backtrack until they find a comfortable pace of progression. The therapist will want to explore the specific details of areas of conflict or anxiety. It may be necessary to shift the entire sequence into low gear and spread the sensate focus exercises over several weeks to months. Once performance anxiety has established a foothold, it can be tenacious. Cooperation, patience, and understanding are a necessity.

Men experiencing performance anxiety and couples whose previously vibrant sex life is now more appropriately described as humdrum generally respond well to the sensate focus exercises. Couples whose sex life is impeded by interpersonal conflict and anger respond poorly or not at all. Depressed men, men with organic impotence, and men who have little or no interest in restoring potency do not respond.

Exercises to Delay Ejaculation

Psychologists and sex therapists cite an 80 to 85 percent success rate in helping men overcome their tendency to ejaculate before maximal sexual excitement has been achieved. Two maneuvers—the squeeze technique and the start-stop technique—help men acquire a sense of confidence and control about timing of ejaculation. Both exercises utilize partner-initiated masturbation to stimulate arousal and are often performed in conjunction with a sensate focus program.

The squeeze technique encourages penile stroking and genital caressing up to the point of orgasm. When the man senses that he is about to ejaculate, he signals his partner, who lightly circles the fingers of her free hand around the glans, the bulbous tip of the penis. When the man senses he has achieved some control of his impulse to ejaculate, stimulation resumes until he reaches a sense of containment of semen.

The start-stop technique also begins with partner-initiated penile stroking to activate an erection. When the man is near ejaculation, he instructs his partner to stop. After a few moments (or minutes) he gives the signal to start, and the process is repeated. As the exercises progress, the interval between the start and stop signals lengthens until finally the man acquires the ability to determine the moment of ejaculation.

The couple may repeat the squeeze or start-stop exercises as often as they like during a session; ultimately, the man will ejaculate. Gradually, as the man becomes used to experiencing prolonged pleasure from sexual stimulation, he will gain confidence and control over the timing of his ejaculation.

Insight Therapy

Impotent men with more deeply rooted emotional problems do not benefit from sensate focus therapy. They must come to terms with the seeds of their discontent through short-term or in-depth therapy. Insight therapy involves an exploration of the factors responsible for original and current erectile failure. The man is obliged to reexamine all aspects of his sexual life.

Andrew's sexual problems began after his forced retirement. He was unable to make love to his wife the night he received the news.

His retirement plan provided a comfortable income but no solace. In his preretirement days he went to bed confident that he would be at work the following morning. Sexual intercourse was never a problem. Now he went to bed worrying not only about the next day but the rest of his life. His morning and nighttime erections were as firm as ever, but he could not muster an erection when he attempted to have sex. He felt like a failure.

The sense of worthlessness engendered by his obligatory retirement was overwhelming, and Andrew plunged himself into a frenzy of activity to reaffirm his value as a man. Unfortunately, the intensity of his activity consumed all of his intellectual and sexual energy, leaving no room for his wife. A realignment of priorities was in order. Andrew was encouraged to restructure his daily activity and carve out a specific time of day to focus some of his considerable energy on his sexual feelings for his wife.

Crises have a way of galvanizing a relationship between caring couples, and Andrew was able to reaffirm his love for his wife and rechannel his energies appropriately so that his erectile function and their sexual happiness were "better than they had ever been before retirement."

All the circumstances surrounding Andrew's sexual problems were of recent onset and readily recalled so that his therapist had little difficulty piecing together the psychodynamics of his impotence and formulating a treatment plan. This is not always the case.

On occasion, the psychologic root cause of impotence is buried deep within a man's subconscious and is revealed through the more elaborate psychiatric probing available only with psychoanalysis.

In 1985 Robert was forty-four, single, and impotent. Married briefly, then divorced, he was something of an enigma: He was healthy, working full-time, and had no difficulty meeting and dating women. Morning erections were normal and he could masturbate, but he was unable to have an erection during sex. When a relationship became serious Robert became emotionally aroused but could not translate this sense of sexual excitement into an erection. Eventually, he became embarrassed and stopped dating altogether.

No clues regarding the origin of his sexual problems were forthcoming from the standard psychiatric interviews. Eventually the psychiatrist suggested psychoanalysis to see if the process of free association would divulge the source of his repressed anxiety about sex.

Psychoanalytic sessions are, by nature, rambling and not immediately productive. However, after several sessions, as Robert was recalling events of his childhood, he blurted out, "Don't pull your pants down. Don't let them see you with your pants down. If you have to pee, make sure no one is looking."

Here was the clue the psychiatrist needed. As a child of two Robert and his family were trapped in Poland during World War II. The father's greatest fear was that because he, Robert, and his brothers had been circumcised, the Nazis would immediately recognize them as Jews. It was for that reason that his father admonished Robert and his brothers never to expose their penises.

Information imprinted in the subconscious of a terrified two-year-old boy is difficult to extricate. It was this fear inculcated in Robert as a youngster that prevented him from undressing as a prelude to having a satisfactory sexual relationship with any women. Only by recognizing and confronting his subconscious fears about exposing his penis was Robert able to feel comfortable and successful in a sexual relationship.

Depression

Depression is different from sadness. We all get periodically despondent, unhappy, and disheartened over life's disappointments. After a period of brooding and feeling sorry for ourselves, we usually resume normal function.

Depression, however, disables a person. People who are depressed frequently feel worthless, helpless, and guilt ridden. They cannot muster the energy, enthusiasm, and concentration needed for most activities, including sex. Impotence, predictably, reinforces the depression.

Depressed people have abnormal sleeping patterns. On the one hand, many depressed people develop insomnia: Either they are unable to drop off to sleep, or they tend to wake in the middle of the night and cannot fall asleep again. On the other hand, a significant number of depressed people sleep far too long and too much, yet still feel fatigued. Depressed individuals may be plagued by a variety of other physical symptoms including headaches, persistent dry mouth, stomachaches, excessive belching, passing wind, occasional palpitations, frequent constipation, and inexplicable weight loss. Symptoms such as these should not be ignored, for they may be harbingers of serious physical problems. However, when medical investigation fails to disclose any physical cause, a diagnosis of depression must be considered.

Health professionals rely on information from patient interviews to establish the diagnosis of depression and then turn to standardized formats like the Hamilton Depression Scale (HAM-D) to gauge the severity of depressive symptoms. The HAM-D explores and grades different aspects of depression, including mood, sleeping problems, feelings of guilt, suicidal thoughts, and sexual dysfunction, and then assigns a numerical score to reflect the intensity of each symptom. The greater the depression, the higher the score. As treatment alleviates depression, HAM-D scores return to normal.

The severity of the depression determines the therapeutic approach. Some depressed men may be incapacitated or suicidal. They may well require hospitalization. Less severely impaired men, who are troubled primarily by their depression-induced impotence and inability to function at work and in relationships, can be treated as outpatients. Generally, treatment involves a combined approach utilizing psychotherapy and antidepressant medication.

A wide range of drugs capable of stabilizing mood and relieving depression are available. The combination of antidepressant medications and psychotherapy is usually effective, and sexual potency frequently returns as treatment lifts the depression.

However, antidepressant medication can create another sexual problem. About 25 to 50 percent of men treated with antidepressants experience some difficulty in ejaculating. This is sometimes overcome by switching to another medication (see chapter 9).

12

Penile Implants

Surgical implantation of penile prosthetic devices is today a commonly accepted means of restoring erectile capability to impotent men. In 1989 U.S. surgeons implanted an estimated 27,500 penile prostheses.

Dr. William Scott of the Johns Hopkins Medical School and Dr. Michael Small, now professor of urology at the University of Miami Medical School, and his associate Dr. H. M. Carrion are recognized as the patron saints of modern penile prosthesis implant surgery. Dr. Scott fashioned an inflatable silicone penile prosthesis (IPP) that he first implanted in early 1973. Drs. Small and Carrion developed their unit shortly thereafter. The Scott and Small-Carrion devices are the prototypes for most of today's penile prostheses.

The original Scott prosthesis, a multicomponent device, had a fluid reservoir implanted in the lower abdomen. A tube from this reservoir was connected to a bulb in the scrotum. The penis remained in a normal flaccid state until intercourse was desired. Then an erection was created by pumping the scrotal bulb to transfer the fluid from the reservoir to the penile implant (see figure 10).

The Small-Carrion prosthesis did not rely on hydraulics to convert the penis from a flaccid to an erect state. Once inserted in the penile corporal bodies, the device provided a perpetual erection. Although highly desirable during moments of sexual intimacy, this proved to be something of a burden at other times. The first recipients of Small-Carrion penile implants found it necessary to gird themselves in tight-fitting underwear or wear baggy pants to camouflage their protruding penis. Concealment was the watchword for these men.

Penile implant surgery has become so popular that in less than fifteen years the procedure has generated its own legacy of legends, mythology, and misconceptions. Since penile prosthetic implants are such an integral component of the current spectum of therapeutic options offered to impotent men, it is important for the potential penile implant recipient to ask the following questions:

- What aspects of sexual function are improved or unchanged following prosthesis implantation?
- What types of prostheses are currently available?
- How are prostheses implanted?
- Are there any complications of prosthesis surgery?
- Am I an appropriate candidate for prosthesis surgery?
- What factors determine patient-partner satisfaction or dissatisfaction following surgery?

Penile prostheses serve only one function: They provide the penile shaft with sufficient rigidity to allow for vaginal penetration. They do not increase penis size, nor do they enhance any other aspect of the male sexual response cycle. One of the common misconceptions about penile prosthetic surgery is that men who receive prostheses will be endowed with a penis of prodigious length and girth. This is not the case. Prostheses cannot lengthen the penis since the rods are inserted in the

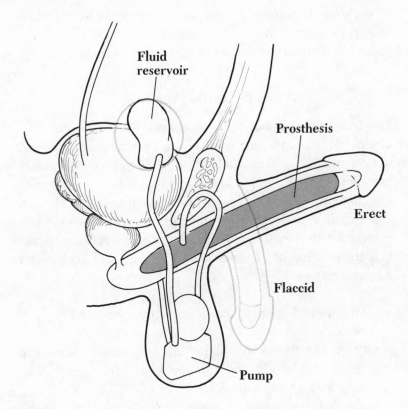

Figure 10.   The multicomponent inflatable penile prosthesis.

corpora cavernosa of the nonerect penis; they must be confined to this limited anatomic space.

In this way the erectile capability created by a penile prosthesis differs from spontaneous erections. The naturally occurring spontaneous erection causes a discernible increase in penile length and girth. The discrepancy between a man's recollection of the size of his prior erections and the erection afforded by the penile prosthesis may cause some disappointment. The prosthetic erection provides only the rigidity needed for penetration, nothing more.

Men with penile prostheses do not experience enhanced arousal, nor do they have any sense of amplified ejaculation or orgasm. Indeed, most recipients indicate that those aspects of sex may be somewhat less satisfactory than before. This disappointment, however, is usually overshadowed by the sheer relief of once again being able to have erections.

Types of Penile Prostheses

The Small-Carrion and Scott penile prostheses are still used but are not the only options. There are a number of different devices on the market today. Four discrete categories of prostheses—semirigid, malleable, inflatable, and hinged—are currently available. All the units listed below have been judged safe and effective by an expert group of urologic surgeons recruited by the American Medical Association to participate in a recent Diagnostic and Therapeutic Technology Assessment panel.

- The original *Small-Carrion* prosthesis consists simply of two rigid rods.
- Penile prostheses with abdominal fluid reservoirs include the *Scott-AMS 700* and a similar device manufactured by the Mentor Corporation.
- The *Jonas* prosthesis is a semimalleable device that depends on a network of internal silver wires to allow for some degree of flexibility.
- The *OmniPhase* and *DuraPhase* prostheses have internal cables that allow the device to bend to a flaccid state when not in use. These units are activated by adjusting the cable to produce penile rigidity. Other malleable devices like the *AMS 600* and *Mentor* have similar designs.
- The *Finney* prosthesis is hinged and converts from flaccid to rigid state merely by locking the hinge in place.
- Newer inflatable prostheses like the *Hydroflex* and *FlexiFlate* have internal fluid systems and are designated as self-contained penile prostheses (SCPP). The SCPP transforms the penis from a flaccid to erect state by manipulation of a valve implanted in the tip of the penis (see figure 11).

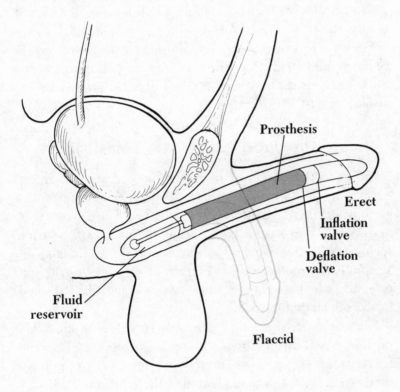

Figure 11.   Self-contained inflatable prosthesis with inflation and deflation valves shown.

Individual urologic surgeons may at one time or another favor one prosthesis over another. However, no single device has yet emerged as the dominant unit of choice. Each device has its own intrinsic advantages and disadvantages (see table 2). The rigid, malleable, hinged, and controlled expansion cylinder devices do not increase penis length or girth. These devices come in a variety of lengths; the urologist chooses from an inventory of prosthetic units a rod customized for each individual patient. The Scott and the comparable Mentor multicomponent inflatable penile prostheses (IPPs) both allow some increase in penile girth and rigidity without changing penis length.

Most urologists take pains to discuss this issue in detail. It is important for potential recipients to understand this pre-operatively lest they harbor any illusions of acquiring significant augmentation of penile anatomy and sexual prowess. Such fantasies can never be fulfilled by any of the currently available prosthetic devices.

How Prostheses Are Implanted

Normal erections occur as increased blood flows into and is trapped in the two corpora cavernosa and the corpus spongiosum. Penile prosthetic devices, whatever kind, all attempt to duplicate this process by outfitting the penis with silicone surrogates for the two corpora cavernosa. (The corpus spongiosum is not replaced during implant surgery.) Prior to implantation, the tissue in the penile cavernosa must be stretched to accommodate the rods.

Patients receiving either the Scott or Mentor inflatable prosthesis require one additional surgical procedure. The bulb for activation or transfer of fluid from a reservoir to the prosthetic shaft is surgically implanted in the scrotum.

Most prostheses are inserted by making a surgical incision either in the lower abdomen or at the junction of the penis and the scrotum and then advancing the rod forward toward the tip of the penis. Some of the newer self-contained penile prostheses, on the other hand, may be inserted by making an incision around the tip of the penis and pushing the prosthetic rods backward toward the bony joint at the end of the torso. The patient usually requires general anesthesia and stays in the hospital three to five days. Some surgeons are giving patients a spinal block (or spinal epidural anesthesia) and sending them home on the same day, but this practice is not widespread. Inflammation, a reaction to the insertion of a foreign body in the penis, causes some postoperative pain, which is controlled by medication. The pain subsides as the inflammation wanes. Following surgery, the patient must allow four to six weeks for healing. During this interval the silicone rods

Table 2. Types of Penile Prostheses

TYPE	NAME	ADVANTAGES	DISADVANTAGES
Rigid	Small-Carrion	Permanent erection	Permanent erection difficult to conceal Penis slips out of vagina during intercourse
Malleable	Jonas Mentor AMS 600	Easy to insert Minimal patient education Relatively inexpensive Adequate rigidity	Penis permanently firm Penile pain Can irritate or rupture the urethra Numbness of glans Failure due to fracture of internal wires
Inflatable: extrapenile fluid reservoir	Scott-AMS 700 Mentor	Attempts to mimic normal erections Adequate rigidity	Frequent mechanical failure requiring reoperation Surgery complex Requires manual dexterity to operate
Inflatable: intrapenile fluid reservoir	Hydroflex FlexiFlate	Readily concealed Adequate rigidity	Requires manual dexterity to operate
Hinged/Segmented	OmniPhase DuraPhase Finney	Surgery not complex Little manual dexterity required Flaccid at rest Adequate rigidity	Does not increase penile length or width

become firmly embedded and anchored in the penile shaft. Then the prosthesis is ready for use.

Success Rate

Recipients of penile prostheses are generally pleased with the results. All acquire a rigidity of the penile shaft adequate for penetration. Initial reports from urologic surgeons were glowing, with success rates reported at 90 to 95 percent. Long-term follow-up has tempered this enthusiasm to some degree. Today, patient and partner satisfaction is closer to 60 to 75 percent.

Complications of Penile Prosthesis Surgery

A surprisingly large number of men will require repeat surgery. The most common complications are mechanical failure of the prosthesis, postoperative infection, and penile pain.

Mechanical complications occur most often in multicomponent inflatable prostheses and reflect malfunction in the workings of the rods, cylinders, or hydraulic system, or kinks in the tubing. The prosthesis must be removed and replaced with either a new, identical unit or an alternative type of prosthesis; the choice is up to the urologist and patient.

Postoperative wound infection is less common today than in the past. Now implant recipients receive antibiotic treatment during and immediately after surgery.

Postoperative pain does occur in some patients. It is usually localized in the tip of the penis (the glans); however, discomfort in the penile shaft, scrotum, base of the penis, or abdomen is not uncommon. In one series of 179 penile prosthesis implants performed at the Mayo Clinic, 61 patients reported complications with the prostheses' mechanisms. Another 42 patients experienced pain, most commonly at the tip of the penis, but occasionally in the penile shaft, scrotum, base of the penis, or abdomen. Of these men, 32 rated their pain moderate or severe.

Pain can herald a more serious problem. It may imply that the position of the prosthesis compromises the function of other vital structures. Pressure on the urethra will cause pain and is a warning of some underlying problem. Paraplegic patients, however, do not perceive pain. As many as one-third of impotent paraplegic men with penile prostheses experience damage to their urethra within six months after surgery.

Research indicates that complications as well as the need for reoperation seem to depend on the type of device implanted, the duration of the follow-up, and the group of patients studied. For example, patients implanted with the older, rigid Small-Carrion prosthesis rarely require reoperation. The reoperation rate is much higher with inflatable penile prostheses (IPP) (see table 3). The malleable and self-contained penile prostheses (SCPP) are the least prone to mechanical breakdown. However, these devices are relatively new, and most urologists have little more than two to three years of experience with them. Still, even within this brief time span, reoperation rates of 14 to 22 percent have been reported.

Table 3. Results of Penile Prostheses Surgery

TYPE	REOP (%)	COMPLICATIONS (%)
Inflatable Penile Prosthesis (IPP)	41	6.8
Small-Carrion	11	10
Jonas	10	7
Self-Contained Penile Prosthesis (SCPP)	18	10

Satisfaction Following Penile Prosthesis Surgery

Although surgical success rates for some devices now approach 90 to 95 percent, patient satisfaction does not parallel this impressive figure. A major problem is disappointment with postoperative penile length and width. Some men never attempt intercourse after the prosthesis is implanted; others have intercourse for only a brief time and then abandon sexual activities. Additional areas of disaffection with prostheses surfaced in response to specific questions.

The majority of urologists are men, and in the beginning the male perspective distinctly covered the reported results of prosthesis surgery. Female health care professionals saw things differently. They approached the issue of satisfaction after implantation by interviewing both partners. Some couples were not having intercourse at all. Of those who were having intercourse, 25 percent reported restriction in positions because of the decreased penis size. Fifteen percent of the men experienced diminution of orgasmic intensity. Still, 79 percent of men said that they would, if given the opportunity, undergo the operation again. Only 59 percent of their partners had no hesitation.

Some urologists claim that satisfaction depends on the type of prosthesis, with IPP recipients being generally more satisfied than those who receive other prostheses. Because they are easily concealed and readily activated, one would have anticipated that the multicomponent IPP would have emerged by now as the dominant, if not the only, penile prosthetic device implanted.

This has not turned out to be the case, for two reasons. Significant problems with the internal hydraulics of IPPs remain, and mechanical failures are common. Perhaps more troublesome is the fact that a certain amount of manual dexterity is required to inflate the IPP.

Originally, in an effort to mimic the genital caressing that is a natural component of sexual foreplay, the man's sexual partner was encouraged to play an active role in pumping the scrotal bulb so that fluid could be transferred from the abdominal reservoir to the prosthesis, a maneuver intended to mimic a stimulated erection. This has not been as warmly embraced as expected.

Sexual partners are often unwilling to participate in the pumping procedure. Some are simply not deft at manipulating the scrotal bulb. As a result, inadequate amounts of fluid are transferred from the reservoir to the prosthesis shaft, and a

suboptimal erection ensues. In such cases failure of the device
has been ascribed not to mechanical problems of the unit itself
but to the inadequate level of participation of sexual partners.
Those who have been unwilling to become involved as vigorous squeezers of the scrotal bulb have been decried as
"timid pumpers." Other factors may also have a significant
impact on postoperative sexual satisfaction. Any of the following put the couple's satisfaction at risk:

- extreme obesity
- psychogenic impotence
- impotence not the only sexual problem
- sexual dysfunction in woman
- severe marital conflict
- unreasonable expectations
- partner opposed to surgery
- woman pressuring man to have surgery
- couple ceased all sexual touching

Obese patients are often displeased following penile prosthesis surgery because the length of the unit protruding beneath their lower abdominal fat pad is limited. Most
prostheses are approximately eight inches in length. If there
is an extensive overhanging fat pad, then perhaps only an
additional four inches of rigid penile tissue will protrude for
purposes of sexual intercourse. If the patient's partner is also
obese, it will be very difficult for the couple to find a position
in which penile-vaginal penetration and adequate vaginal containment is possible. For obese couples, postoperative sexual
gratification may be limited.

Inappropriate expectations are high on the list of reasons
for postoperative patient/partner dissatisfaction. The prosthesis provides only the penile rigidity necessary to achieve
vaginal penetration. Patients who anticipate that the equip-
ment will allow them to recapture the real, or imagined, sexual
prowess of their youth are likely to be displeased.

Patients whose impotence is attributed to psychogenic factors do not derive as much long-term benefit from prosthetic surgery as those whose impotence is caused by either neurogenic or vasculogenic factors.

On occasion, impotent men have sexual problems other than erectile dysfunction. Lack of spontaneous arousal, limited libido, and ejaculatory disorders are not corrected by penile prosthesis implantation.

The level of preoperative patient/partner interaction is a critical determinant in evaluating postoperative satisfaction. If, for example, the female partner has her own sexual dysfunction, such as pain during intercourse, then she may be fearful of experiencing vaginal penetration again. A man may choose to have a penile prosthetic implant without notifying his partner. Such a decision is commonly interpreted as a rejection of the partner. In addition, some women are fearful that their previously impotent partners, now outfitted with penile prostheses, will seek other lovers. Limited studies exploring this question have indicated that penile prosthesis recipients are no more susceptible to seduction, nor do they routinely seek out new sexual opportunities more often than other comparably aged potent men.

On the other hand, some female partners of impotent men, frustrated after long periods of sexual abstinence, may pressure the men into surgery. Any discordance in patient/partner desires for penile prosthesis surgery is considered a major risk factor for postoperative dissatisfaction.

Couples who have distanced themselves sexually from each other and have ceased hugging, touching, and all sensual and erotic contact may not be able to retrieve all aspects of normal sexual function merely by placing a prosthetic rod in the penis. Clearly, satisfaction is maximal only when both partners are involved in all discussions and decisions from the beginning.

Candidates for Penile Prosthesis Surgery

Prostheses have been implanted in men with virtually every known type of impotence, but some men are more appropriate candidates for surgery than others. Urologic surgeons prefer to implant devices in men whose impotence is a result of a physical cause, either neurogenic or vasculogenic. Included in the category of neurogenic impotence are men with diabetes mellitus, spinal cord injuries, and multiple sclerosis; paraplegics; and men whose pelvic nerves have been damaged or severed during prostate or lower abdominal surgery. Vasculogenic impotence applies to men with either decreased penile arterial inflow or increased venous outflow; vascular surgery is the preferred form of treatment for these men. But they are not always willing to go through the somewhat more complex surgical procedures and may elect prosthetic implantation instead.

As noted, patients with Peyronie's disease have no difficulty achieving an erection. But the erection bends, so the penis deviates, often creating a J-shaped erection unsuitable for intercourse. Peyronie's disease occurs when fibrous bands grow in the outer lining of the penis and tug at the penile shaft. The bands can be removed surgically, but this is only a temporary solution because these strictures tend to recur at the same or different locations in the penis. Implanting a prosthesis is often the only way to circumvent the problem.

Men with endocrine disorders, whose potency can be restored with appropriate hormonal therapy, and men with overt psychological problems, who require psychotherapy, psychiatric medications, or both, are the only groups to whom physicians do not routinely offer penile prosthetic implants.

The Future of Penile Prosthesis Surgery

The initial brouhaha attending the introduction and early years of penile prosthesis surgery has subsided. It is now possible to reflect and cast a sober eye on the role of penile prostheses in the treatment of impotent men. It is clear now that surgical skills alone are not enough to solve the problem of impotence.

The penile prosthesis industry is highly lucrative and competitive. The five penile prosthesis manufacturers collectively account for $60 million in worldwide sales. Penile prosthetic surgery is expensive. The cost of the prosthesis, hospitalization, and urologic surgeon's fees can be as high as $10,000 to $12,000. This figure is applicable to those men who have their surgery and three to five days of postoperative care in the hospital. Most medical insurance plans cover the cost of surgery only for patients with documented organic impotence. With improved anesthetic skills and pressure to cut down on the high cost of hospitalization, some urologists have been experimenting with same-day ambulatory outpatient surgery. It is too early to determine whether this novel approach will safely replace the more traditional three-to-five-day hospitalization.

13

Penile Injection

Puncturing one's penis with a needle is not for the squeamish. Piercing the penis with a needle and then injecting a chemical to enhance one's sexual potency sounds more like a bizarre, sadomasochistic nightmare from the annals of Krafft-Ebing's *Psychopathia Sexualis* than a doctor-recommended treatment of impotence. Nevertheless, many men, with guidance from their physicians, practice self-injection of the penis to achieve an erection. Three types of medications—phentolamine (an alpha-blocker), papaverine (a smooth-muscle relaxant), and prostaglandin E_1—are used.

These medications are effective in stimulating erections because they overcome neurologic signals that normally keep the penis in a limp or flaccid state. Neurologic control of erections is vested in the sympathetic nervous system.

To understand how the sympathetic nervous system works, it is useful to create a simple scary example. Imagine that you are alone at night walking down a dark street. There is no sound. Then, as you are absorbed with your thoughts, someone sneaks up behind you and says, "Boo!"

Your sympathetic nervous system immediately swings into action to cause, among other reactions, an increase in pulse rate and blood pressure. The change in pulse and blood pressure is caused by internally produced adrenalinelike compounds with unique properties designated alpha or beta. Beta forces cause an increase in pulse rate, while alpha influences are responsible for the increase in blood pressure.

What does this have to do with erections? The penis is richly endowed with extensions of the sympathetic nervous system, specifically nerves of the alpha type. Alpha influences play a vital role as facilitators or inhibitors of normal erections.

When the alpha forces dominate, the penis remains at rest. A penile injection of a medication that blocks the alpha nerves overrides these influences and makes it possible for a full and unrestrained flow of blood to be directed into the erectile bodies of the penis. Medications like phentolamine, an alpha-blocker, and prostaglandin E_1, a muscle relaxant with probable alpha-blocking activity, cause erections by interfering with the prevailing nerve signals that would maintain the penis in a limp state.

It is somewhat more difficult to understand exactly how papaverine works. There are no papaverine receptors in the penis. Papaverine, unlike alpha-adrenergic compounds or prostaglandins, is not made by the body. However, papaverine has one characteristic that is useful in inducing an erection: It is a *smooth*-muscle relaxant.

The body has two types of muscles, striated and smooth. Striated muscles are literally striped in appearance and are, for the most part, under voluntary control. The muscles of the arms, legs, and face are striated muscles. Smooth muscles are not under volitional control. For example, the muscles in the intestines are smooth muscles. The muscles lining the penile blood vessels that must dilate for an erection to occur are also smooth muscles. It is presumed that papaverine induces an erection by causing these intrapenile smooth muscles to relax, thereby allowing or encouraging increased blood flow into the penis.

To be fully effective, the medications must be injected directly into one of the penile erectile bodies, the corporus cavernosum (see figure 12). (The medication will diffuse over to the other side of the penis so that symmetrical erection is acquired.)

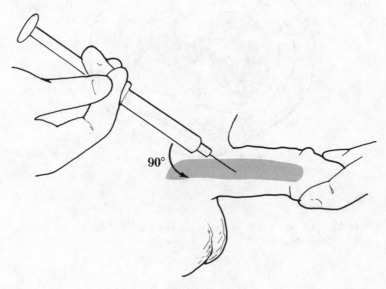

Figure 12.   Method of intrapenile injection.

A cross section of the penis illustrates the corpora cavernosa surrounded by the thick outer fibrous sheath (tunica albuginea) (see figure 13). The needle is inserted at a ninety-degree angle to the penile shaft and must penetrate the tunica albuginea to make contact with the corpus cavernosum. Patients are taught to advance the needle into the penis and wait for a slight "give" in the resistance. When they sense this change in tension, they know that they have punctured the tunica albuginea. The medicine is then injected. An erection occurs within ten to thirty minutes. Most urologists recommend that injection be performed no more than twice a week.

Papaverine, phentolamine, and prostaglandin E_1 (marketed as alprostadil [Prostin VR Pediatric]) are available in most pharmacies, as are insulin syringes with very small needles.

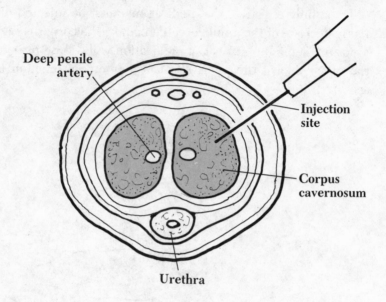

Figure 13. Cross section of the penis showing the thick outer lining (tunica albuginea) surrounding the corpora cavernosa.

Candidates for Intrapenile Injections

Sixty-five to 75 percent of impotent men can have an erection induced by the intrapenile injection of combined papaverine and phentolamine. Preliminary reports from Japan suggest that 86 percent acquire erections with prostaglandin E_1 alone. The men most likely to respond to injections are those with neurogenic impotence. Injection can induce erections in men with vasculogenic impotence, but only if the dose of medication is significantly greater than that needed for other men. Intrapenile injections are not an effective long-term treatment for men with vasculogenic impotence because the injections will eventually fail to stimulate erections even if a large amount of drug is used. In addition, for reasons that remain unclear, about one-third of men with psychogenic impotence do not respond adequately to intrapenile injections.

Patient and Partner Satisfaction

More than half of the patients enrolled in one penile injection program reported that they were either "very satisfied" or "satisfied" with the program; one-third considered the treatment "not acceptable." Men seem more pleased than women with penile injection programs. They describe an increase in erectile function, intercourse frequency, and improved self-image.

Some women note that they are turned off by the artificiality of the procedure. On the other hand, some get into the spirit of things; one said, "When I'm in the mood I simply leave a syringe on the pillow and he gets the message."

Seven years after the first intrapenile papaverine injections were given, doctors have enough experience to recognize that this form of treatment is not a panacea. Specific problems reported include lack of a sustained erectile response over time, high patient drop-out rate, and complications.

Different doses of drugs have been administered. Doses effective in inducing the first erection are not consistently effective in maintaining satisfactory erections with each successive injection. A need to increase the dose after a while or switch from one medication to another seems to be standard. Even men who have a fully satisfactory response do not always stay with this form of treatment; about one-third drop out.

Complications

Three different complications have been attributed to intrapenile pharmacotherapy: penile nodules and sclerosis, abnormalities of liver function, and prolonged erection (or priapism).

Men who continue to inject papaverine/phentolamine develop nodules along the shaft and scarring in the body of the penis. To date, nodules have not developed with prostaglandin E_1 injections, but problems may surface as physicians and patients gain more experience with the drug.

It was originally believed that papaverine or papaverine/ phentolamine injected directly into the penis would remain there and not enter the bloodstream. This has proved not to be the case. Some of the mixture enters the general circulation and causes damage to the liver. Up to 40 percent of men who continue long-term treatment can expect to develop at least one abnormality of liver function: mild inflammation. Liver function tests return to normal when treatment stops. Prostagladin E_1, however, is fully metabolized in the penis and does not circulate.

From the very beginning it was apparent that some men who injected papaverine were susceptible to prolonged erections lasting for six to twelve hours. The prospect of a twelve-hour erection may, at first, tantalize some men with fantasies of nonstop, daylong fornication. However, men who have chemically induced prolonged erections know that this is not possible. Prolonged erections are often extremely painful and hence neither sexually exciting nor erotic.

Prolonged erections were most commonly observed in men with neurogenic impotence. This is truly unfortunate. There is no way of restoring the nerve connections to the penis that have been severed as a result of spinal trauma, diabetes mellitus, or pelvic surgery. However, penile anatomy and blood supply remain intact. Intrapenile papaverine injections seemed an ideal solution for these men. Men with neurogenic impotence do achieve a most dramatic and prompt restoration of erectile function after the first papaverine injection. The problem is that they are too responsive, which makes them so susceptible to priapism.

Mindful of this, physicians have been adjusting the treatment schedules to lower the dose of papaverine and phentolamine. Papaverine doses initially calibrated at 80 milligrams are now down to 25 milligrams or less. Still, problems with priapism persist.

Priapism is a medical emergency and requires immediate intervention. An erection that persists beyond six hours deprives penile tissues of adequate oxygen. Without sufficient oxygen, penile tissue deteriorates. Reversal of priapism usually requires the intrapenile infusion of additional chemicals to counteract the effect of papaverine or phentolamine. Often this treatment alone allows blood to drain from the penis.

Surgery is required for those men whose priapism remains even after medical treatment. On occasion, Draconian surgical maneuvers have been necessary to decompress the swollen penis and reverse the erection. Some patients have had major distortions in penile anatomy, and many have been left permanently impotent.

Those men unfortunate enough to have experienced these severe reactions have sought redress. Their attorneys have initiated litigation against the physicians who recommended participation in the penile autoinjection program in the first place and the Eli Lilly Corporation, the pharmaceutical company that manufactures and distributes injectable papaverine.

Upset that papaverine had caused serious patient disability and corporate liability, Lilly rewrote its package information form to express displeasure at the use of its medication for purposes of inducing a penile erection. The current package insert provided with each vial of papaverine now states the following under the "contraindications" section:

> Papaverine hydrochloride is not indicated for the treatment of impotence by intracorporeal injection. The intracorporeal injection of papaverine hydrochloride has been reported to have resulted in persistent priapism requiring medical and surgical intervention.

This disclaimer shifted the onus of continued use of papaverine for intracorporeal injection away from the manufacturer and squarely on the shoulders of the prescribing urologist and his or her patients. This action did not, however, sound a death knell for all intrapenile injection programs.

All three medicines work, but no single drug or combination of drugs has yet to merge as the treatment of choice. In comparison studies of intrapenile injections of papaverine, papaverine/phentolamine combination, and prostaglandin E_1 given to the same impotent men, the papaverine/phentolamine combination and prostaglandin E_1 were clearly superior and roughly comparable. Differences between the two surfaced when the number and types of complications were examined.

Whereas none of the men who received prostaglandin E_1 experienced prolonged erections, 7 to 10 percent of those taking the papaverine/phentolamine combination did. This finding should have allowed prostaglandin E_1 to emerge as the drug of choice. Unfortunately, 19 percent of men injected with prostaglandin E_1 experienced a painful erection.

There is one overriding problem plaguing enthusiasts of intrapenile injection for the diagnosis and/or treatment of impotence. Not one of the drugs currently employed has been approved for this use by the FDA. The manufacturers of papaverine include a specific warning *against* its use for purposes of inducing an erection. Prostaglandin E_1 is approved only for the treatment of a rare form of congenital heart disease in newborn infants.

The lack of government and pharmaceutical approval has disappointed, but not deterred, urologists. According to published reports, as of December 1989, more than 4,000 men in the United States, Europe, and Japan have participated in intrapenile injection programs and received a total number of injections in excess of 60,000. Urologists who have been at the forefront of research are convinced that this treatment is both safe and effective. They claim to be puzzled by the recalcitrance of the FDA and comparable foreign governmental agencies to approve the continued use of intrapenile pharmacotherapy for impotent men. Their puzzlement is disingenuous.

FDA approval has not been forthcoming because the pharmaceutical companies that manufacture papaverine (Eli Lilly) and prostaglandin E_1 (Upjohn) have not asked for FDA approval. Upjohn has made a corporate decision not to invest the time and money needed to obtain FDA approval of intrapenile prostaglandin E_1 injections as an accepted treatment of impotence. Unlike Eli Lilly, Upjohn has not, however, issued a statement discouraging the use of its product for treatment of impotence. Intrapenile pharmacotherapy with papaverine, phentolamine, or prostaglandin E_1 now has the dubious distinction of being the most widely recommended but still unapproved treatment of impotence.

14

Other Therapies

Impotence has plagued mankind for thousands of years. The distress caused by this symptom has provided the stimulus for the development of a series of innovative and ingenious treatments designed to allow men to recapture sexual vigor. Some therapies have evolved as spin-offs of sound scientific research. A few trace their origins to traditional folk remedies; many "guaranteed cures" turn out to be hoaxes. Today the impotent man is offered an extraordinary range of therapeutic options, quite literally running the gamut from A (aphrodisiacs) to Z (zinc). Bringing up the end of the therapeutic alphabet are vacuum devices, vitamin E, yohimbine, and zinc.

The Vacuum Constrictor Device (VCD)

Any system encouraging blood to flow into and be captured in the penis should produce an erection. This is the principle behind the vacuum constrictor device (VCD) now offered as a noninvasive means of restoring erections for some impotent men.

Devices resembling the VCD have been shuttling in and out of favor for more than seventy years. The original concept has been traced to the inventor Otto Lederer, who in 1917 was granted a patent for a unit that would allow "persons considered completely impotent to perform sexual intercourse in a normal manner." It is not known whether the Lederer device was ever produced. A newer product, undoubtedly a variation on the original theme, was developed by a man to help him deal with his own impotence. It is marketed under the name ErecAid and sells for about $400.

There are several components to the ErecAid device (see figure 14). A cylinder designed to fit over the limp penis is connected to a hand-operated vacuum pump. Suction from the pump creates a negative pressure within the cylinder, and this encourages an increased flow of arterial blood into the penis. Venous outflow is prevented by tight bands that fit over

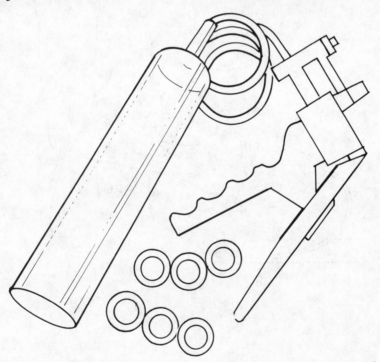

Figure 14. Vacuum chamber and bands used to achieve an erection with a vacuum constrictor device.

the base of the penis. A petroleum jelly–like substance lubricates the system and seals the base of the cylinder. When a user achieves an adequate erection (and with the rubber bands inhibiting venous outflow still attached), he removes the cylinder. The vacuum-induced erection is maintained for up to thirty minutes.

Some dexterity and skill are required to operate the VCD. The user must place the unit on some nearby surface while the limp penis is stuffed into the vacuum chamber. With the penis and the chamber perched at an angle, his hands are free to pump air out of the chamber and affix the restraining bands to the base of the penis (see figure 15). Often, significant pres-

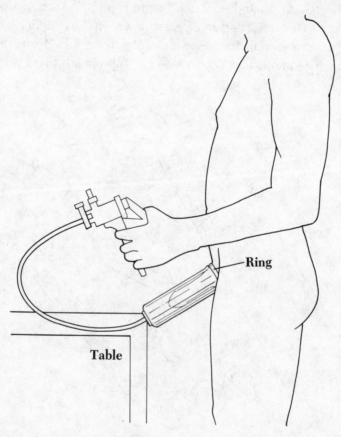

Figure 15. Proper positioning of patient and VCD prior to initiating a vacuum-induced erection.

sure must be applied. Three to seven minutes in the vacuum chamber are required to achieve erections of optimum rigidity.

Limitations of the VCD

Not only does vacuum-induced pressure in the VCD cause most men to experience penile discomfort, but the erection achieved by this means is inferior to a spontaneous erection in three significant aspects. Once the erection has been induced by the vacuum, the rubber bands in place at the base of the penis choke off blood flow into the penis. This causes penile skin temperatures to fall to 96°F. One-third of the female partners of men using VCDs found the chilled penis displeasing during intercourse.

Another drawback is that as the penis becomes engorged and congested by the VCD-induced suction and inhibition of venous outflow, penile circumference increases more than it would during a normal erection. This gives the penis a sausagelike appearance.

Third, the erection created by the VCD is rigid only from the point at which the rubber bands are affixed. This means that it is not fully upright and rigid like a normal erection, but flexible and capable of swiveling or pivoting at its base.

The VCD also does not permit normal ejaculation. Because the rubber bands remain in place throughout the sexual act, semen is trapped in the urethra and can be released only after the bands are removed.

Despite these limitations, the manufacturers of the VCD say that more than 15,000 units have been sold in the United States since 1983.

Reports on Patients' Experiences

Objective evidence regarding the effectiveness of the device is scanty. There are only a few reports in the medical literature, most by Dr. Perry Nadig, a urologist from San Antonio, of positive VCD experience. One English urologist evaluated the VCD in ten impotent diabetic men who used the unit for three months; they all found it fully satisfactory and were able to have intercourse on the average of six times a month.

Dr. Nadig's experience with the VCD is the most extensive. His first report, in the early 1980s, described the responses of thirty-five impotent men using the VCD in his clinic. Twenty-seven achieved an erection of sufficient length, girth, and rigidity for intercourse. An additional five experienced some increase in penile length, but rigidity was considered inadequate for intercourse. Twenty-four of them continued to use the device.

By 1989 Dr. Nadig could report on the experiences of 340 impotent men who had used the VCD. Eighty-nine percent achieved erections satisfactory for intercourse. Eighty-one percent purchased a VCD for use at home, and of those who used the unit, most were said to be "satisfied and continued to use the VCD regularly." Dr. Nadig was frank about side effects, including fainting (three cases), infection of the foreskin (one case), and penile pain (most of the men).

Initial interpretation of questionnaires prepared and distributed by the manufacturer of the VCD unit suggests that although 92 percent of men maintain they can achieve a satisfactory VCD-induced erection, only 75 percent continue to use the device. These men limit intercourse to about once every two weeks, perhaps because of side effects or mechanical problems.

Pain and discomfort were common experiences. Black-and-blue marks on the penis occurred in almost all the men. All respondents indicated that they needed a considerable amount of practice time to learn how to use the unit, and once they had acquired the skill to use it, the interval from initiating vacuum suction to the development of an erection ranged from thirty seconds to more than seven minutes and averaged about two and a half minutes.

Only 57 percent of patients rated their orgasm as pleasant; 9 percent described pain; and 12 percent were unable to ejaculate at all.

A Marginal Treatment

Urologists are not keen on recommending the VCD. At present, inadequate independent data are available to assess the role of the vacuum devices in the overall treatment of impotence. Further, some men should not use the VCD: Those who are receiving anticoagulant or aspirin treatment are susceptible to extensive intrapenile bleeding when the device is applied. Men who are at risk for the development of priapism, such as those with sickle cell disease and leukemia, are cautioned not to use the unit.

It is clear that some men are delighted with and continue to use the VCD to induce an erection. However, in the absence of other corroborating data, the VCD must be classified as a treatment of marginal value at best.

Vitamin E

Vitamins are chemical substances ingested in the diet that are essential for the normal operation of the metabolic machinery that drives our internal systems. Inadequate vitamin intake leads to symptoms of vitamin deficiency. For example, lack of vitamin C produces scurvy, and diets deficient in vitamin A cause night blindness.

Doctors became fascinated with vitamins because men and women seem to require such minuscule amounts of these substances to remain free of disease. As each new vitamin was discovered, scientists rushed to their laboratories to discover its precise function. To do this they fed experimental animals diets deficient only in that single vitamin.

The initial studies of vitamin E were carried out in the early 1920s. Male rats fed a vitamin E–deficient diet became sterile. These rats remained potent, however, and could have erections and mount a receptive female rat. But somehow this aspect of the research was overlooked. By convoluted reasoning the illusion emerged that vitamin E was important not only for rodent sperm production, but also somehow enhanced male sexual potency. This misconception has been readily, indeed ardently, embraced by the public. Manufacturers of vitamin E have done nothing to dispel this notion.

Rats and humans are quite different. Vitamin E has been administered to men suffering from infertility and impotence and has been ineffective in reversing either condition.

Despite this overwhelming evidence, the public seems to want to believe that vitamin E has aphrodisiac qualities. Fortunately, vitamin E is relatively innocuous and has been consumed without any ill effect. The same cannot be said for other alleged aphrodisiac drugs.

Yohimbine

Man has always been intrigued and tantalized by the fantasy of discovering an aphrodisiac, a substance that would stimulate his sexual appetite and power. Some foods and drugs are thought to be imbued with aphrodisiac properties, and those who were privy to the secret ingredients of the sexually stimulating substances were highly valued. The physician to Louis XIV slipped the monarch a special potion each night before the king received a new lady in his bedchambers. The royal physician's potions were not always effective, causing the king to become displeased, truculent, and vengeful.

At one time it was believed that the drug yohimbine had aphrodisiac properties. Certainly yohimbine had the appropriately exotic lineage to satisfy preconceptions of what an aphrodisiac should be. Yohimbine was derived from the bark of a tree that grows only in Africa. It was believed that natives boiled the tree bark in a caldron and then harvested the residue. The yohimbine extract was then administered to men and women who were said to experience a sudden and striking increase in sexual desire.

Intrigued by these descriptions, Western scientists decided to look into the effects of yohimbine in man. Yohimbine, marketed under the name of Afrodex, was tested in 10,000 impotent men. Eighty percent were said to have restoration of potency. That report was published in 1968. Immediately thereafter Afrodex vanished.

Interest in yohimbine was resurrected in the 1980s. Yohimbine, now available as the prescription drug Yocon, has been tested in one hundred impotent men. Half received yohimbine and the other half placebo. Twenty-one percent of the yohimbine-treated patients had a complete return of sexual function. A surprising 13.8 percent of placebo-treated patients also reported a full return of sexual function. Statistical analysis indicated that yohimbine was not significantly better than placebo in restoring potency.

Was it possible that the dose of yohimbine administered was too low to have produced a positive effect on male sexual function? Apparently not. Larger doses of yohimbine were given in another study involving eighty-two impotent men. With higher doses 14 percent reported a full return of sexual function. This figure is roughly comparable to the 13.8 percent full response in the placebo-treated patients in the prior study.

Yohimbine is an intriguing drug because it functions as an alpha-adrenergic antagonist. Drugs that block the action of alpha-adrenergic nerves have been successful in inducing erections, but only when injected directly into the penis (see chapter 13). The specific subset of alpha-adrenergic properties needed to induce an erection is unfortunately missing in yohimbine. The alpha-adrenergic properties retained by yohimbine cause blood pressure and pulse to rise, and provoke a sense of nervousness and anxiety.

Current studies indicate that yohimbine is no more successful than placebo in restoring sexual function. Yohimbine has worrisome cardiovascular side effects. Placebos do not.

Zinc

The importance of zinc in the reproductive process has assumed legendary, almost mythical proportions. Today, zinc acetate tablets are commonly recommended as a nostrum to improve flagging sexual prowess and restore fertility.

Much of our early knowledge of zinc deficiency was derived from studies in mice and rats. Weanling rodents fed a zinc-

deficient diet develop testicular failure and suffer growth re-
tardation.

Zinc is essential in man. Fortunately, it is ubiquitous, and
spontaneous zinc deficiency is uncommon. Zinc deficiency occurs predominantly in extreme-starvation states in the Third
World. In this country zinc deficiency can be detected in black
males with sickle cell anemia and in men and women with
chronic kidney disease. Some poorly nourished alcoholics also
have inadequate zinc in their systems. Unfortunately, zinc
therapy has not yet proven to be effective in restoring potency.

15

Male Fertility
and Infertility

The most accurate recent surveys indicate that 8.6 million couples in the United States would like to, but cannot, have children. They are said to be involuntarily infertile. In 40 to 50 percent of the cases a "male factor" is considered to be wholly or partially responsible for the couple's sterility. The term *male factor* is appropriately vague, for it encompasses a spectrum of disorders disrupting the natural sequence of events leading to sperm-ovum fusion. To understand how this might occur it is necessary to examine the individual events in the reproductive process.

Normal Fertility and Fertilization

During ovulation, one egg (ovum) is released into one fallopian tube, where fertilization occurs.

A man's fertility depends upon his ability to generate millions of sperm daily. Although only one sperm is necessary for fertilization, the odds against insemination are formidable. To improve chances for conception, the system is flooded with sperm. During sexual intercourse several million sperm are deposited in the vagina. Many perish immediately in the hostile acid environment of vaginal fluids. Others die at the cervix, the entrance to the womb.

Freshly ejaculated sperm can swim, but they cannot fertilize: They are buffeted by a sea of fertility-impeding chemicals called decapacitating agents. To acquire full fertilizing capability sperm must be transformed or capacitated. Normally this occurs as sperm pass through the uterine cervix. Capacitated sperm then swim through the uterus at a steady pace, destined for the woman's fallopian tube. The sperm must arrive in time to fertilize her recently ovulated ovum. There is only a limited window of opportunity for fertilization, thirty-six hours each month.

When sperm enter the fallopian tube, they veer like a heat-seeking missile, aiming for the ovum. Immediately prior to the moment of fertilization sperm go through yet another transformation, referred to as hyperactivated motility, in which they shift from a smooth gliding swimming pattern to a rapid corkscrew flailing motion with high torque. Enzymes contained within the sperm head then disperse the shroud of cells (cumulus oophorus) surrounding the ovum and bring the sperm in direct contact with the outer lining of the ovum (zona pellucida). Additional sperm enzymes are released so that the sperm can burrow into the zona pellucida and gain access to the body of the ovum (ooplasm). It is in the ooplasm that the union of sperm and ovum nucleus takes place finalizing the act of fertilization.

The process of fertilization, though intricate and complex, functions quite satisfactorily for the majority of men and women. Healthy couples conceive at a predictable rate of 20 percent per month. After one year of "unprotected" intercourse (that is, intercourse without contraception), 86 to 90 percent of all normal couples will have initiated a pregnancy. Those who are unable to conceive after one year are considered to be infertile.

Invariably it is the woman who first seeks help to determine why she cannot bear children. When an evaluation indicates that she is ovulating normally, has normal female anatomy, and no obvious impediment to conception, suspicion is cast on the male partner.

The man is considered responsible for the infertility if the sperm he produces are few in number, unable to swim with proper velocity, immobilized by his partner's cervical mucus (and unable to enter her womb), or incapable of surviving the trek from vagina to fallopian tube.

Normal Sperm Production

As noted, there is a division of labor within the testicles: Leydig cells produce testosterone, and Sertoli cells manufacture sperm. Two pituitary hormones oversee testosterone and sperm production. Luteinizing hormone (LH) activates Leydig-cell testosterone production, whereas follicle stimulating hormone (FSH) supervises sperm production. The relationship between the pituitary hormones and the testicle is one of mutual dependence. The testicle relies on the pituitary to provide LH and FSH. The pituitary, in turn, releases these hormones in response to the productivity of the cells of the testicle.

When testosterone output lags, blood testosterone values fall. These low testosterone levels goad the pituitary into dispatching additional LH to increase the supply of testosterone. In addition to sperm, the Sertoli cells manufacture a protein called inhibin. If sperm production fails, inhibin levels decline. In response to low inhibin levels, the pituitary releases more FSH in hopes of revitalizing sperm output.

There is, unfortunately, a point of no return. Occasionally the testicles are so wracked by infection or inflammation that they cannot mobilize enough healthy Sertoli cells to rejuvenate sperm production even in response to a surge in FSH. Then sperm counts remain low and FSH levels high. The level of FSH circulating in the blood is a reliable index of the extent of damage suffered by the sperm-producing Sertoli cells. A combination of a low sperm count and elevated serum FSH level bespeaks a poor prognosis for resurrecting sperm development. In contrast, low sperm count with normal or low FSH levels indicates opportunities for improving sperm output with hormone therapy.

Because of the prodigious obstacles to fertilization, nature has provided man with the ability to produce millions of sperm. Exactly how many millions are needed to guarantee fertility has been a subject of some debate. Scientists have recently learned that it is not merely the total number but also the shape, swimming velocity, and maturity of sperm that determine fertility. These vital properties of sperm are revealed by an examination of the semen.

Semen Analysis

The semen analysis is the linchpin in the evaluation of the infertile man. This microscopic study, performed after men provide semen by masturbating, provides valuable information about the total number of sperm present, how many are freely moving (the motility index), and how long their active swimming motion persists.

By convention, sperm counts are recorded as millions of sperm per one cubic centimeter (cc) of semen. Normal fertile men have a sperm count of between 20 and 80 million sperm/cc. Although some men with sperm counts as low as 5 to 10 million/cc have been able to impregnate their partners, 20 million sperm/cc is considered the minimal number required for fertilization.

Some men have no sperm in their ejaculate, a condition referred to as azoospermia. The problem usually results from testicular failure due to either viral injury such as mumps or genetic disorders such as Klinefelter's syndrome (see chapter 8). Occasionally, the testicle produces a normal amount of sperm, but none appears in the ejaculate because the ducts carrying sperm from the testicle to the urethra are blocked. This condition is called obstructive azoospermia.

Some men produce some, but not enough, sperm and are said to have oligospermia. This problem can be a consequence of an intrinsically imperfect testicle or an impairment in the pituitary stimulus to sperm development. Differentiating testicular (primary) from pituitary (secondary) causes of oligospermia is of paramount importance. When the testicle's sperm-producing cells are scarred, sperm production cannot proceed or be activated. However, if these cells are not producing sperm only because of the lack of proper hormonal stimulation, opportunities exist for increasing the testicle's sperm output.

A substantial number of infertile men have normal numbers of sperm (they are referred to as "normal but infertile"). Immunologic factors, antisperm antibodies, or sperm-cervical mucus incompatibility are thought to be responsible for their infertility.

Curiously, one group of infertile men makes too many sperm, a condition known as polyzoospermia. Infertile polyzoospermic men have mind-boggling sperm counts of 250 million/cc. Approximately 38 percent of them can initiate a pregnancy, but unfortunately, the sperm-ovum union is often blighted. The partners of polyzoospermic men suffer a high incidence of first-trimester miscarriage; the factors responsible remain obscure.

Routine semen analysis also provides information regarding the swimming velocity of sperm. Sperm have a tail that moves back and forth to propel the sperm in seminal fluid and through the vagina, womb, and ultimately into the fallopian tubes. Some sperm are simply better swimmers than others. Examined under the microscope, healthy sperm exhibit an effortless swimming (or motility) pattern that ordinarily persists for several hours. Defective sperm have a languorous or sluggish swimming motion. They lack the vigor to make the journey to inseminate an egg. Men whose sperm concentration is dominated by a high percentage of languid sperm are infertile. The technical name for this condition is asthenospermia.

Infections of the prostate gland, seminal vesicles, or urethra cause bacteria and pus (white blood cells) to mingle with sperm. Bacteria and pus disrupt sperm motility and diminish fertilizing capacity. This condition, called pyospermia, can be treated with antibiotics. Once the infection is cleared up, sperm swim more freely, and opportunities for fertility are enhanced.

Treatment of Infertility

The treatment of male infertility is, in principle, simple: First pinpoint and then correct the impediment to fertility. Scientists have devised a legion of medical and surgical programs to encourage a man's testicles to increase their output of sperm, to enhance and invigorate sperm's fertilizing capability, to counteract the immunologic barriers to conception, to unclog channels blocking the unrestrained flow of sperm from the testicle to the urethra, and to bypass anatomic obstacles to insemination.

No Sperm: Azoospermia

If repeated semen analyses fail to show sperm in semen, the diagnosis of azoospermia is secure. The outlook for the azoospermic man is not hopeful unless the cause can be traced to a defect in pituitary gland stimulation to the testicle or an obstruction in one of the ducts responsible for transporting sperm from the testicle to the seminal fluid.

Men whose testicles are understimulated by the pituitary can be treated with synthetic pituitary hormones. In cases of obstructive azoospermia, microsurgery can alleviate the obstruction and allow sperm to flow freely from the testicle to the urethra.

Unfortunately, the majority of men with azoospermia have irreparable damage to their testicles. Included in this group are men whose Leydig cells (testosterone secretion) and Sertoli cells (sperm output) never functioned properly because of genetic disorders. They are impotent as well as infertile. Another group of men have suffered a selective injury to their sperm-producing Sertoli cells. Since their Leydig cells churn out normal amounts of testosterone, these men remain potent. But they are infertile because their Sertoli cells were harmed by viral infections, chemotherapy, or X-ray treatments. There is no way to revive sperm production once the Sertoli cells are fatally injured.

Low Sperm Count: Oligospermia

Men with low sperm counts (oligospermia) may not be, strictly speaking, infertile, but subfertile. Fertility is not always an either/or phenomenon. Some subfertile men are capable of initiating a pregnancy, but not within the same standard one-year time frame; it takes two to three years of unprotected intercourse.

In many cases, the number and quality of sperm produced by a man's testicles can be improved either by varicocele surgery or by the administration of hormones or drugs.

The Varicocele and Varicocele Surgery

Surgical treatment is predicated on the assumption that the testicles are intrinsically capable of normal sperm production but are restrained from doing so by a local structural abnormality. A tangle of veins, a varicocele, may surround the testicle (usually the left one). Most varicoceles are readily apparent to sight and touch (see figure 16). Men with varicoceles frequently have semen analyses characterized by low sperm counts or a disproportionate number of poorly swimming sperm.

The current thinking is that the heat generated by blood in the varicocele has a negative impact on the testicle's ability to produce sperm. Varicocele surgery allows testicular temperatures to return to normal, and if there are no other obstacles, normal sperm production and fertility should be the outcome. Several studies have compared the pregnancy rates of

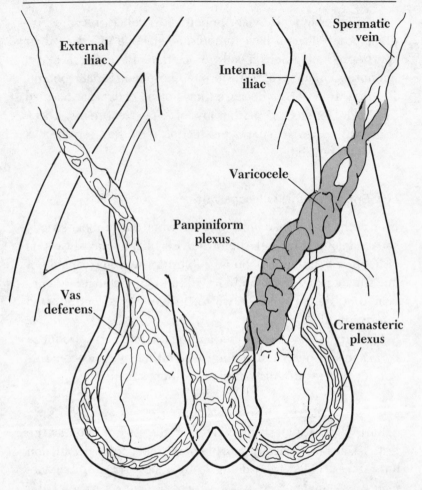

Figure 16.   Testicle with varicocele (in black) adjacent to left testicle.

women whose partners had varicocele surgery with those of women whose partners did not have surgery to correct the problem. The results are inconclusive. Men who do not have varicocele surgery may be no less fertile than men who undergo surgery. Since these men are not truly infertile but merely subfertile, their partners would likely conceive eventually without surgery.

Men considered the best candidates for varicocele surgery are under thirty years old, have reductions in sperm count to no less than 10 to 15 million/cc, may have a decrease in testicular size (but only in one testicle), have no evidence of pus in their semen, and have normal or only slightly elevated FSH levels. Men unlikely to benefit from surgery are over thirty-eight years of age, have sperm counts lower than 5 million/cc, frequently have decreased volume of both testicles or pus in their semen, and have a markedly elevated serum FSH value indicating severe damage to the sperm-producing Sertoli cells.

Hormone and Drug Treatments

Hormone and drug treatments are designed to provide supplemental stimulation to the sperm-producing Sertoli cells in the testicles. Serum FSH levels before treatment provide a useful index of subsequent success. Only men with normal or just slightly elevated serum FSH levels are appropriate candidates.

Several forms of treatment—all of them arduous—are available. The most elaborate option is reserved for men with idiopathic hypogonadotropic hypogonadism (see chapter 8). A pump, identical to an insulin pump, links up with a tube and needle to deliver intermittent pulses of gonadotropin releasing hormone (GnRH) into the bloodstream. This stimulates pituitary release of both LH and FSH. The impact of LH is seen immediately: Pulses of LH invigorate testosterone production. Serum testosterone, libido, and potency increase, although sperm production initially remains low. With time, the sperm-producing cells start to respond, and sperm counts increase after nine to twelve months of therapy.

Increasing the pulsatile release of LH and FSH can also be accomplished with clomiphene (Clomid, Serophene), an oral medication commonly used to treat infertility in women. Clomiphene increases the frequency and amplitude of LH and FSH pulses and stimulates testosterone and sperm production in some men. Sperm count does not increase until the patient has had six to nine months of therapy. Although clomiphene has been employed for many years to increase sperm output, it is not yet sanctioned for this use by the Food and Drug Administration (FDA).

Oddly enough, two female hormones have proved effective in increasing sperm production. A substance normally produced during pregnancy—human growth chorionic gonadotropin (hCG)—has LH-like properties and stimulates testosterone production. Human menopausal gonadotropin (hMG) (found in an equally unlikely source: the urine of menopausal women), has potent FSH-like properties and can also increase sperm output.

Both hCG and hMG must be administered by injection. The usual procedure is to start treatment with hCG to increase the testicles' output of testosterone. The resulting high testosterone levels can reawaken dormant sperm-producing cells. This alone may be a sufficient stimulus to start up sperm production again. In other instances, men may need additional hormonal stimulus in the form of the FSH surrogate hMG.

Injections of hCG are given twice a week for three to six months. If sperm counts show no improvement, hMG injections are added to the treatment schedule. Patience and forbearance are required. Improvements in sperm output can be provoked with this form of therapy, but they occur only after nine to fifteen months of therapy.

Incompatibility of Sperm and Cervical Mucus

Men with normal sperm counts, the "normal but infertile" group, require investigation beyond the semen analysis. If a man's sperm output is adequate, and his sperm motility is vigorous, additional studies must be performed to address the specific issue of why his apparently healthy sperm do not inseminate.

In many cases, it is the inability of sperm to penetrate cervical mucus that is causing the infertility. The mucus produced by a woman's cervix is, for most of the month, impervious to sperm. The character of the mucus changes—it becomes pliant to allow sperm to gain safe passage into the uterus—only in the middle of the menstrual cycle, during ovulation. Swimming sperm linger for a time in the cervical mucus before they tunnel through into the uterus. This temporary stopover has provided investigators with another research tool, the postcoital test.

This test has now become an important component of the evaluation of infertile couples with unexplained infertility. Two to four hours after intercourse, the woman comes to the doctor's office. The physician takes a sample of her cervical mucus and examines it under the microscope. The presence of actively swimming sperm is normal. If sperm are present but not actively swimming, a "sperm-cervical mucus incompatibility" is thought to be the cause of the infertility.

Once the postcoital test determines that sperm are present but immobilized by cervical mucus, further sophisticated tests are required to resolve whether the cervical mucus or the sperm is causing the problem.

Samples of the cervical mucus are exposed to sperm from a male known to be fertile. (The test is done on a slide in the physician's laboratory.) If the stranger's sperm swim easily through the cervical mucus, the mucus is not the source of the problem. If, on the other hand, the foreign sperm make no headway or are immobilized by the cervical mucus, a "cervical factor" must contribute to the couple's infertility.

In the second experiment, the man's sperm and cervical mucus from a woman known to be fertile are combined. If the sperm are incapable of making progress through the cervical mucus, it is presumed that the sperm possess antibodies that preclude penetration of any cervical mucus. This condition, known as "immunologic infertility," occurs in about 8 percent of infertile men.

Immunologic barriers to fertility are found more frequently in men who have had vasectomies. Vasectomized men who divorce or lose their wives to illness may remarry and wish to reconsider the wisdom of their self-imposed sterility. A vasectomy reversal operation (vasovasotomy) is possible. Following vasovasotomy, normal numbers of sperm appear in the semen, but in 60 to 80 percent of cases the sperm are coated with an antibody and neither penetrate cervical mucus nor fertilize ova. Neutralizing the fertility-impeding impact of this antibody is essential if fertility is to be restored.

Treatment of Immunologic Infertility

The cortisonelike medications prednisolone and prednisone, with their potent antibody-neutralizing effects, are the mainstay of treatment of immunologic infertility.

Intensive prednisolone therapy (about 96 milligrams daily) is prescribed for the man during the two weeks preceding his partner's ovulation. The prednisolone should neutralize, or inhibit, all the antibodies residing on the surface of the sperm head. Sexual intercourse is timed to coincide with ovulation, at which time prednisolone is discontinued. If the woman does not become pregnant with the first course of prednisolone therapy, subsequent cycles can be initiated.

On the average, 35 percent of couples infertile because of immunologic infertility can expect to initiate a pregnancy after prednisolone or prednisone treatment. Some men respond more satisfactorily to treatment than others. Men who have been infertile for two years or less are more likely to respond to prednisolone than those with long-standing infertility. The treatment achieves optimum results when the woman's physiology offers no impediment to fertilization. Women who have anatomical abnormalities of the uterus or fallopian tubes or a "cervical factor" that impairs the passage of sperm into the uterus must be treated along with their partners.

This form of therapy is not benign. Prednisolone and prednisone can cause acne, weight gain, headaches, upset stomach, and especially mood swings. Men taking high doses of prednisolone have insomnia and are irritable, aggressive, and argumentative. These consistent and predictable side effects reverse fully when treatment ends.

Noncoital Reproduction

It is now possible for men and women to initiate a pregnancy without even engaging in sexual intercourse. This is referred to as noncoital reproduction. Two generic classes of noncoital reproduction are currently available: artificial insemination of the women with either her partner's or a donor's sperm and assisted reproduction such as in vitro fertilization and gamete intrafallopian tube transfer.

Artificial Insemination

Artificial insemination is a viable treatment option for some infertile couples. The man's sperm can be collected and infused directly into the woman's vagina. To improve opportunities for insemination, the collected sperm can be processed and treated (capacitated) so that only the most actively swimming and viable sperm are used. In cases of cervical factor infertility, the physician can bypass the cervix by instilling the sperm directly into the uterus.

Artificial insemination with the partner's sperm is successful in inducing a pregnancy in only about 18 percent of infertile couples. Researcher's believe the low success rate is due to the fact that the sperm are most likely flawed and burdened by an inherent defect in fertilizing potential. Current methods of sperm enrichment enhance the fertilizing capability of these sperm only to a limited degree.

Statistics improve if artificial insemination is performed with normal sperm. Young men with certain types of malignancies such as lymphoma, Hodgkin's disease, and testicular cancer often have normal sperm production. Remarkable advances in medicine have allowed many of these men to be cured. However, as noted, the drugs and X-ray treatment commonly used invariably cause irreparable damage to sperm-producing cells. Prior to treatment, men can collect semen by masturbation, deposit it in a sperm bank, and preserve it for future use.

After the cancer victim has been successfully treated, he now has the opportunity to start a family. Young men with cancer who make a "deposit" in the sperm bank prior to chemotherapy can anticipate a 45 to 60 percent chance of pregnancy when they make a "withdrawal" and use their own sperm to inseminate their partners.

Insemination with donor sperm has produced successful

pregnancies in a quarter of a million Americans. The sperm donor, usually a healthy young medical or graduate student, provides semen for a fee and is guaranteed anonymity. He will not know the woman to be inseminated, and she in turn will be unable to determine his identity. The doctor performing the insemination attempts to match general physical appearance between the donor and the woman's husband.

Insemination coincides with the women's ovulation. Several monthly inseminations are often required before pregnancy is established. Donor insemination succeeds 60 to 75 percent of the time, depending on the woman's age and regularity of ovulation. Age is a critical factor. In one large study performed in France, pregnancy rates were 74 percent in women under thirty, 61 percent in women between thirty-one and thirty-five, but only 53 percent in women over thirty-five.

Inseminated pregnancies are indistinguishable from spontaneous pregnancies in terms of rates of miscarriage (15 to 18 percent) and birth defects (4 to 5 percent).

In Vitro Fertilization

In women with blocked fallopian tubes, the egg cannot migrate into the fallopian tube to be available for insemination. A procedure has been developed to overcome this anatomic obstacle. The woman takes medication to encourage ovulation of multiple eggs (ova), and then a physician removes the ripened ova directly from the woman's ovary. The ova are placed in a laboratory dish (a petri dish, not a test tube).

The man provides sperm by masturbating. Sperm are first capacitated and then added to the ova. Fertilization and early embryonic development take place in the laboratory dish while hormone treatment prepares the lining of the woman's uterus. Ordinarily several of the growing embryos are implanted in the uterus in the hopes that one or two will survive to term. This procedure is known as in vitro fertilization (IVF).

The same methods have been useful in the treatment of certain infertile men as well. Men with low sperm counts, poor sperm mobility, or normal sperm counts but immunologic infertility have participated in IVF programs.

IVF is beneficial for these men for several reasons. The methods used in preparing sperm for IVF act as a gleaning process and salvage only the most motile and fertile sperm. Men with low sperm counts occasionally have limited numbers of perfectly normal sperm. These healthy sperm are usually overlooked in a semen analysis dominated by languid sperm. A medical laboratory can selectively segregate the handful of active sperm from their more inefficient brethren and then treat this elite corps further to allow them to undergo the process of capacitation, enhancing their fertilization potential.

The anatomic barriers to sperm-ovum interaction that may be present in men with immunologic infertility are obliterated by the simple expedient of placing the enriched sperm in direct contact with ova. The total number of sperm that must be present for IVF is only a fraction—one-tenth—of that required for insemination through intercourse. The success rate—pregnancy culminating in a live birth—is 18 to 28 percent in couples with male factor infertility.

Gamete Intrafallopian Tube Transfer

Fertilization normally takes place not in a laboratory dish but in the fallopian tube. Some individuals have modified the fundamental techniques used in IVF to mimic the normal process of conception. This technique, referred to as gamete intrafallopian tube transfer (GIFT), has been especially useful in the treatment of infertile men.

As with in vitro fertilization, the woman is treated with hormones to maximize ovulation. Several ova are then removed from her ovary, mixed with the man's capacitated sperm, and inserted back into the fallopian tube. This allows conception to take place within the fallopian tube, mimicking the normal process. The embryo(s) then migrate into the uterus and develop normally (see figure 17).

To date, 18 to 38 percent of couples considered infertile because of a male factor have been able to initiate a pregnancy with GIFT. Additional studies will have to be performed to determine whether this extraordinary success rate can be sustained.

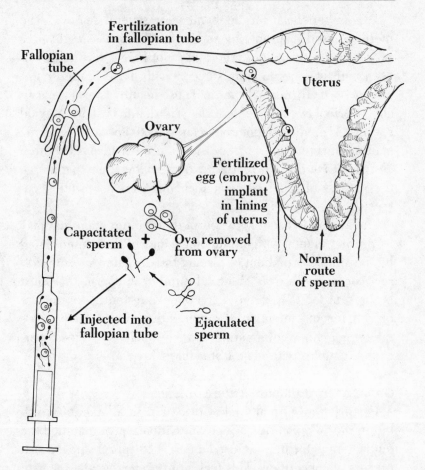

Figure 17.   The GIFT procedure for treatment of infertility: (A) ova retrieved from ovary; (B) ejaculated sperm are capacitated; (C) capacitated
sperm are mixed with ova and injected into the fallopian tube; (D) fertilization takes place in the fallopian tube.

Ethical Issues

Advances in assisted or noncoital reproduction have proceeded at a dizzying pace. The arena, once the exclusive do-
main of infertile couples and their physicians, has now
attracted the attention of religious leaders, laypersons, legis-
lators, and ethicists.

There is, to be sure, something eerie about how facile we have become in tinkering with sperm and ova, as if they were little more than reproductive spare parts. The new technology has offered scientists unprecedented opportunities to examine nuances of reproduction in exquisite detail but has also created unimagined moral dilemmas.

No one quibbles with the propriety of using a husband's sperm to inseminate his wife. Even the use of donor sperm for insemination has now been accepted. But what about donor ova?

The woman participating in an IVF program knows that the hormone treatment she receives will force her ovaries to release up to eight to ten mature ova. This is more than enough for her immediate needs. Ordinarily only three or four ova will be inseminated, allowed to develop into embryos, and then implanted in her uterus. What is the proper disposition of her "surplus" ova? Should they be discarded? Is it preferable to have them fertilized by her husband's sperm, allowed to develop as embryos, and then frozen to be retrieved for use by the couple at a later date? Should unfertilized ova or embryos be donated to other infertile couples?

The American Fertility Society (AFS) has grappled with many of these ethical concerns and has proposed a set of guidelines for donor insemination and IVF. The guidelines suggest that ova and embryos be considered the property of the genetic parents who alone may decide on their disposition. The donation of unused, unfertilized ova as well as early embryos is acknowledged as an acceptable and ethical practice.

Not everyone is comfortable with this formulation. Some religious groups are uneasy with the entire process of assisted reproduction, which they perceive to be "unnatural." Others, willing to accept the principles of IVF, are troubled by unforeseen difficulties that are implicit, if not explicit, in the document as drafted.

The stipulation that the embryos are the "property of the donors" sounds admirable, but what if a husband and wife divorce? Who owns the embryo, husband or wife? What happens if both husband and wife die? Who determines the fate of the orphan embryo? Judges have already been pressed into service to resolve these thorny issues.

IVF and GIFT programs, once restricted to academic centers, are now sprouting as self-contained outpatient facilities. The proliferation of IVF units, some more successful than others, has brought this new reproductive technology within reach of most infertile men and women in this country. Now is the time to reflect on these vexing questions and decide how the new reproductive technology can best be used to the benefit of infertile couples and society.

16

Is There
a Male Climacteric?

The notion that man, as he ages, must inevitably fall prey to a condition analogous to the female menopause has been bandied about for decades. The term *male climacteric* has found favor as the androgynous counterpart to menopause. Male climacteric has been vigorously championed, as if some cosmic fairness doctrine demanded that both men and women experience equal-opportunity afflictions of aging. Others have been just as ardent in insisting that there is no evidence for the existence of a male climacteric.

What Is a "Climacteric"?

Menopause and climacteric are words of Greco-Roman origin. The words *mens* (Greek) or *mensis* (Latin), meaning "month," serve as the root used to designate different stages in the onset (menarche), continuation (menstruation), and cessation (menopause) of monthly cycles of vaginal bleeding.

The word *climacteric* has an equally intriguing linguistic history, dating back to the sixth-century Greek philosopher

Pythagoras. He considered the first climacteric to be at age seven; additional climacterics, pivotal events in a man's life, occurred at ages twenty-one, forty-nine, fifty-six, and eighty-one.

Today, climacteric is used to designate physical changes at different ages in either sex, or in the female as a synonym for menopause. Physicians groping for a succinct phrase to describe the impact of aging on older men found the term *male menopause* unwieldly and biologically silly. Therefore they resurrected the gender-neutral climacteric.

Dr. August Werner, a St. Louis internist, introduced the term *male climacteric* in a medical paper published in 1939 in the *Journal of the American Medical Association.* He thought it was "reasonable to believe that many if not all men passed through a climacteric period somewhat similar to that of women." He described two middle-age men, both of whom we would today recognize as having hormonal deficiencies. Treatment with testosterone injections was said to be beneficial.

Five years later, a burgeoning medical literature on the male climacteric had been amassed. Two physicians, Dr. Carl Heller of Vancouver, Washington, and Dr. Gordon Myers of Detroit, pooled their collective experience and cataloged the symptoms thought to be characteristic of the male climacteric: "nervousness, psychic depression, impaired memory, inability to concentrate, easy fatigability, insomnia, hot flashes, periodic sweating, and loss of sexual vigor." (These symptoms often accompany menopause in women.) They also observed that in contrast to women, these men retained their fertility and experienced no change in secondary sexual characteristics.

Drs. Heller and Myers sensed that psychological factors might be responsible for climacteric symptoms in some men, whereas other men clearly experienced an unequivocal impairment in testicular function as they aged. Their postulate was not fully explored at the time because only primitive diagnostic methods were available in 1944.

Today we have a greater appreciation of the extraordinary

and intricate matrix of internal chemical events that governs our sexual function throughout life.

The Role of Hormones in Sexual and Reproductive Function

From conception to senescence, a single remarkable system, the hypothalamic-pituitary-gonadal axis, masterminds the sexual and reproductive destiny of both men and women (see chapter 8). Individual components of this system, though anatomically remote, must function in a tightly coordinated pattern to ensure the efficient evolution of the species. This axis is active throughout life but is programmed to function at quite different levels of intensity in the developing fetus, childhood, adolescence, peak adult reproductive years, and old age. The system is activated shortly after conception and continues to function throughout our lives, though at varying intensities.

Effects of Aging on Hormonal Production in Women

As women age, their ovaries fail and can neither release ova nor produce the ovarian estrogen hormones. In an effort to resurrect flagging ovarian function and restore estrogen levels to normal, the hypothalamus becomes wildly active, sending bursts of GnRH to the pituitary, which responds by releasing exorbitant amounts of the pituitary hormones LH and FSH.

A normal ovary would respond to these stimuli by increasing estrogen production. The aging ovary is, however, incapable of further hormone production. Thus, serum estrogen levels remain low. (It is these bursts of pituitary gonadotropins working alone or in the presence of a failing ovary that are believed to be responsible for the flushing and sweating that are so characteristic of the hot flashes.)

Effects of Aging on Hormonal Production in Men

Aging men do not experience a comparable drastic decline in the secretion of the testicular hormone testosterone or a dramatic increase in the levels of LH and FSH. However, a man does not escape unscathed from the aging process.

Impact on Testosterone Production

When scientists first looked into the effect of aging on male gonadal hormone secretion, their studies yielded conflicting results. One group found that older men, like older women, experienced a form of gonadal failure. Their testes did not function adequately and were unable to produce normal amounts of either testosterone or sperm. Other investigators presented compelling evidence that aging impairs neither testosterone secretion nor sperm production. There is a reason for this contradiction: Although investigators from both camps set out to examine the same problem, they did not study precisely similar groups of men.

Dr. Alexander Vermeulen, a Belgian scientist, was one of the first to report that a progressive decrease in serum testosterone levels occurred in men after age fifty. He found that men age twenty to fifty had roughly comparable serum testosterone levels. Between the ages of fifty and sixty, levels fell, but only slightly. Then, with each subsequent decade, levels fell markedly. Dr. Vermeulen was careful to note, however, that although serum testosterone levels declined, they didn't reach clinically significant subnormal values until after age eighty.

These observations were supported by a large study of 466 Australian males age two to 101. Again, a progressive decline in serum testosterone levels seemed to be a natural consequence of advancing age, and the report confirmed the older men maintained their serum testosterone levels in the normal range until the eighth decade.

Both studies, as well as comparable reports from the United States, were completed in the mid-1970s, just before gerontology became a full-fledged medical specialty.

When gerontologists began to study the impact of aging on serum testosterone levels, they found quite different results. One group based in Baltimore and another in Boston found that serum testosterone levels did not change with age. Indeed, the values of men age sixty-four to eighty-eight were indistinguishable from those of men age thirty-one to forty-four.

The gerontologists had recruited and studied only extraordinarily healthy older men and women. The gerontologists charged that the earlier reports showing a decrease in serum testosterone levels with age were flawed because the health of the individuals studied was not adequately defined. Many illnesses common to older men can cause serum testosterone levels to fall.

Whenever the conventional wisdom established by one group of researchers is challenged, science benefits. A new flock of scientists now focused their efforts on exploring the impact of aging on male sexual and reproductive function. Dr. Vermeulen, too, extended and expanded his research activities.

Stung by criticism that his earlier observation that decreasing testosterone levels were due to either environmental factors or unrecognized medical problems in the men he studied, Dr. Vermeulen now studied Trappist and Benedictine monks. Once again he found a difference in serum testosterone levels between men under sixty (average age, thirty-seven) and men over sixty (average age, seventy-one), but this time the variation was less pronounced. Although the difference was statistically significant, both values fell well within the normal range for healthy men.

Dr. Vermeulen extended his studies to a larger group and compared the hormone levels of younger and older men living in different environments. His younger group included military draftees and medical workers. Older men were either retired and living at home or were less vigorous nursing-home residents. This time less dramatic decreases in serum testosterone levels were noted. Even men with an average age of ninety-three had testosterone levels in the normal range.

This impressively documented report demonstrated that men experience an ebbing, but no abrupt cessation, of testicular testosterone production with advancing age. Thus, the male situation is not analogous to menopause.

Impact on the Hypothalamic-Pituitary-Gonadal Axis

In the mid-1980s scientists started to tease apart the elements of the driving force behind man's sexual and reproductive life and examine in detail the impact of aging on the components of the hypothalamic-pituitary-gonadal axis system. First, they studied the effect of aging on the hypothalamus alone. Second, they explored the capability of the aging pituitary to respond to hypothalamic signals. Finally, they reevaluated the capacity of the aging testicle to manufacture testosterone and produce sperm.

Results of these carefully crafted studies demonstrated that neither the hypothalamus nor the pituitary nor the testicle works with the same degree of vigor and efficiency in aging men. The differences are subtle and can be discerned only with elaborate and intricate research techniques.

The rhythms governing male sexual function originate in the hypothalamus. A young man's hypothalamus releases GnRH in a brilliant burst, and small blood vessels carry it to the pituitary in a dramatic fanfare. The older man's hypothalamus retains the ability to manufacture and secrete GnRH, but the pulses seem more measured and somewhat less urgent, so that the GnRH signal received by the pituitary is best described as sotto voce.

In younger men, testosterone levels show a distinct rhythmic pattern with highest values in the morning and significantly lower levels in the evening. Older men lose this rhythm, maintaining a constant level of circulating serum testosterone throughout the day. It is as if the driving force regulating sexual function has shifted from high to low gear.

The pituitary can function only when it receives the appropriate GnRH signals from the hypothalamus. As one might anticipate, the dampened pulses of GnRH evoke suboptimal release of pituitary hormones.

The testicle has two biologic functions: to produce the hormone testosterone and to manufacture and release sperm. Different cells in the testis regulate these individual functions. It has been known for some time that the total number of testosterone-producing cells decreased with age. The testicles of older men have at least 44 percent fewer testosterone-producing cells than the testicles of younger men. Older men also have a selective scarring of the sperm-producing cells. Nevertheless, the testicles have an extraordinary reserve capacity and do not need their full complement of cells to function normally. Men who have lost one testicle to surgery maintain testosterone production and full potency and fertility as well.

Does increasing age alone cause a meaningful impairment in testosterone- and sperm-producing capabilites? One obvious way to answer this question is to study these specific components of testicular function in men of advanced age.

A group of physicians from the Max Planck Institute in Germany compared the testicular function of twenty-three men age sixty to eighty-eight with that of twenty men age twenty-four to thirty-seven. First they examined blood samples to determine the levels of the critical hormones testosterone, LH, and FSH. In both groups the levels were normal—and virtually identical. Then they performed sperm counts. The semen analyses of young and old men were similar; both groups' values fell in the normal range considered acceptable for fertility. Finally they examined the fertility potential of these sperm. They found that the sperm of men in the older group (average age, sixty-seven years) had a fertilizing effect equivalent to that of the sperm of men in the younger group (average age, twenty-nine).

A Reappraisal of the Male Climacteric

The incidence of sexual dysfunction in the aging male is high. What is responsible for this?

Probably the best way to understand the impact of aging is to reexamine the symptoms originally thought to be characteristic of the "male climacteric syndrome": nervousness, psychic depression, impaired memory, inability to concentrate, easy fatigability, insomnia, hot flashes, periodic sweating, and loss of sexual vigor.

- Nervousness and depression are most likely a reflection of a bona fide depression that commonly occurs in older men. Treatment is available.
- Memory and concentration problems are probably indications of the mild memory deficit (dementia) that is seen in some, though not all, aging men. Treatment is not yet fully effective.
- Insomnia is also common. The reasons for altered sleep habits are not entirely clear, but it appears that with aging, men and women establish different sleep patterns and require less sleep than they did in their youth. A specific type of insomnia, the inability to stay asleep, may also be a sign of an underlying depression.
- Hot flashes and sweating are relatively uncommon in older men. However, men who have had surgical removal of their testes experience hot flashes.
- Loss of sexual vigor is a common problem for men as they age. The diminution in sexual desire and potency is only occasionally the result of hormone failure. More often a sexual slowing down can be attributed to a combination of physical problems that occur as a natural consequence of aging.

Although all systems required for normal male sexual function remain operational in older men, these systems function with decidedly less verve. With aging, blood flows less briskly to the genitals. Nerves that carry signals to allow erections to occur transmit their impulses with less velocity. The hormonal system that propels male sexual and reproductive function continues to chug along at an adequate, if not ideal, pace. For many older men, the function of vascular, neurologic, and hormonal systems, though suboptimal, is still sufficient for enjoyment of sex.

Thus, it is not the collapse of any single system but rather the collective impact of "adequate but suboptimal" functioning of all three systems that explains the decline in sexual activity.

Unlike the situation in menopause in which a single organ, the ovary, fails, no single organ or system failure can be identified in the aging male. Therefore, strictly speaking, men do not experience anything comparable to menopause; there is no evidence of male climacteric.

For the majority of healthy older men, sexual function persists, but with some limitations:

- Men's ability to experience an erection in response to visual images or fantasy declines with age. Men retain their interest in, and can experience pleasure from, sexual activity but are dependent on more primitive reflexes to acquire an erection.
- The older man retains the ability to have reflex erections in response to manual or oral stimulation. This implies that the local nerves and arteries responsible for providing increased blood flow to the penis are preserved.
- Older men find that their reflex erections do not have the same staying power as the erections they had when they were younger. Continued genital stimulation can extend the duration of the erection.
- Diminished ejaculatory volume is a natural consequence of aging and should not be a cause for concern. Actually, the sperm concentration increases as the volume of fluid declines.

A new term, *presbyrectia,* has been coined by Dr. Helen S. Kaplan of Cornell Medical School in New York to describe the modifications in penile erectile response now accepted as normal for aging men. As presbyopia describes aging men's visual

alterations and presbycussis their decrease in hearing, so presbyrectia characterizes the changing pattern of erectile capability.

It is not possible to assign a precise date for the onset of
presbyrectia for all men. The earliest signs probably surface
sometime after the age of sixty. The process accelerates during
the seventies and is firmly entrenched after the age of eighty.

No one has yet identified a scheme or treatment program
to stave off the inevitable and universal impact of different
stages in the evolution of presbyrectia.

Older men can anticipate that aging will impose some limitations in sexual capacity. Patterns of sexual activity will have
to be realigned to compensate for these limitations. Increasing, almost exclusive, reliance on genital stimulation to initiate
reflex erections is necessary.

Aging itself does not obliterate sexual urges or the ability
to derive pleasure from sex. Couples who work within the
boundaries of sexual functioning imposed by the effects of
aging can continue to experience a satisfying sexual life.

Afterword

An increasing number of health care professionals stand ready to help men with sexual problems. The previously bleak therapeutic landscape is now populated by psychiatrists, psychologists, sex therapists, urologists, and endocrinologists. Each specialist has his or her own unique perspective on the factors responsible for impotence. Their range of therapeutic options is also determined, and to an extent limited, by their perception of the most likely causes of impotence.

Urologists, for example, are surgeons with a particular understanding of male genital anatomy. They are likely to think of impotence as a penile problem. Restore penile rigidity, and potency is restored.

Urologists can provide penile prostheses and instruct men in the proper use of intrapenile injections. Some urologic surgeons, along with their colleagues in vascular surgery, have become skilled in the art of reconstituting vascular channels either to enhance blood flow into, or delay the exit of blood out of, the penis.

Psychiatrists, psychologists, and sex therapists believe that the view of impotence as a problem of penile malfunction is too narrow. They see sex as an interactive phenomenon between two caring people, and believe that the dysfunctional man can recapture his natural sexual feelings and function only by understanding the emotional setting in which sexual problems develop and persist.

Endocrinologists are fascinated by the recent unraveling of details on hormonal regulation of sexual function. They tend to view sexual problems as a breakdown in hormonal linkages within the body; once hormonal problems are identified and treated, sexual function can return.

The availability of so many health care professionals willing and able to help can be both reassuring and bewildering to the impotent man and his partner. Where do they turn first?

Probably the best place to start is with a primary care physician, a family practitioner or internist who has at his or her disposal enough experience and knowledge to start the diagnostic process. Today's primary care physician commonly encounters men with sexual problems and has found ways to help, and may be able to provide complete diagnosis and treatment on his or her own. Or the physician can make an intelligent decision on which subspecialist will best serve the patient's needs.

The urologist, psychiatrist, psychologist, and endocrinologist will review the findings of the primary care physician, propose some more definitive tests, and then recommend an appropriate course of action. The impotent man and his partner should weigh each recommendation carefully before deciding how to proceed. Before deciding on one therapeutic alternative or another—vascular surgery or penile injection or prosthesis, for example—the patient and his partner should be sure that all diagnostic avenues have been adequately explored and discuss the benefits and drawbacks of the recommended treatments.

Fortunately, medical science now has many methods for dealing with male sexual dysfunction. Impotence need not be a lifelong sentence to celibacy; difficulty with conceiving need not condemn a couple to childlessness. Certainly no treatment is foolproof. Nevertheless, if a couple can take that difficult first step to seek help and then communicate openly about the options they have, the results—potency, a satisfying sex life, and, if desired, fertility—can bring good health and well-being.

References

Chapter 2. You Are Not Alone

Frank, E., C. Anderson, and D. Rubinstein. Frequency of sexual dysfunction in "normal" couples. *N. Engl. J. Med.* 299 (1978): 111–15.

Kinsey, A. C., W. B. Pomeroy, and C. E. Martin. *Sexual behavior in the human male.* Philadelphia: Saunders, 1948.

Moore, J. T., and Y. Goldstein. Sexual problems among family medicine patients. *J. Fam. Pract.* 10 (1980): 243–47.

Reading, A. E., and W. M. Wiest. An analysis of self-reported sexual behavior in a sample of normal males. *Archives of Sexual Behavior* 13 (1984): 69–83.

Slag, M. F., J. E. Morley, M. K. Elson, et al. Impotence in medical clinic outpatients. *JAMA* 249 (1983): 1736–40.

Spector, K. R., and M. Boyle. The prevalence and perceived aetiology of male sexual problems in a non-clinical sample. *Br. J. Med. Psychol.* 59 (1986): 351–58.

Werner, A. Sexual dysfunction in college men and women. *Am. J. Psychiatry* 123 (1975): 164–68.

Chapter 4. Defining the Problem

Cole, T. M. Sexuality in the spinal cord injured. In R. Green, ed. *Human sexuality: a health practitioner's text.* Baltimore: Williams and Wilkins, 1975.

deGroat, W. C., and A. M. Booth. Physiology of male sexual function. *Ann. Int. Med.* 92 (1980): 329–31.

Friedman, M. Success phobia and retarded ejaculation. *Am. J. Psychother.* 27 (1973): 78–84.

Levine, S. B. Marital sexual dysfunction: ejaculation disturbances.
Ann. Int. Med. 84 (1976): 575–79.

Ovesey, L., and H. Meyers. Retarded ejaculation: psychodynamics
and psychotherapy. *Am. J. Psychother.* 22 (1968): 185–201.

Sadock, V. A. Normal human sexuality and psychosexual disorders. In H. I. Kaplan and B. J. Sadock, eds. *Comprehensive text-
book of psychiatry,* 4th ed. Baltimore: Williams and Wilkins,
1985.

Silver, J. R. Sexual problems in disorders of the nervous system. I.
Anatomical and physiological aspects. *Br. Med. J.* 3 (1975): 480–
82.

Chapter 6. The Impulses for Potency: The Nervous System

Allen, R. P., and C. B. Brendler. Nocturnal penile tumescence pre-
dicting response to intracorporeal pharmacological erection testing. *J. Urol.* 140 (1988): 518–22.

Benson, G. S., J. McConnell, and L. I. Lipshultz. Neuromorphol-
ogy and neuropharmacology of the human penis. *J. Clin. Invest.*
65 (1980): 506–13.

Brindley, G. S. Physiology of erection and management of paraplegic infertility. In T. B. Hargreave, ed. *Male infertility.* Berlin:
Springer-Verlag, 1983.

Condra, M., A. Morales, D. H. Surridge, J. A. Owen, P. Marshall,
and J. Fenemore. The unreliability of nocturnal penile tumescence recording as an outcome measurement in the treatment of
organic impotence. *J. Urol.* 135 (1986): 280–82.

Doman, J., and D. J. Kupfer. Computer analysis of EEG, EOG,
and NPT activity during sleep. *Int. J. Biomed. Comput.* 23 (1988):
191–200.

Ellis, D. J., K. Doghramji, and D. H. Bagley. Snap-gauge band
versus penile rigidity in impotence assessment. *J. Urol.* 140
(1988): 61–63.

Goldstein, I., M. B. Siroky, D. S. Sax, and R. J. Krane. Neuro-
urologic abnormalities in multiple sclerosis. *J. Urol.* 128 (1982):
541–45.

Kaiser, F. E., and S. G. Korenman. Impotence in diabetic men.
Am. J. Med. 85 (1988): 147–52.

Kaneko, S., and W. E. Bradley. Penile electrodiagnosis. Value of
bulbocavernosus reflex latency versus nerve conduction velocity
of the dorsal nerve of the penis in diagnosis of diabetic impotence.
J. Urol. 137 (1987): 933–35.

Karacan, I., P. J. Salis, M. Hirshkowitz, R. E. Borreson, E. Narter, and R. L. Williams. Erectile dysfunction in hypertensive men: sleep-related erections, penile blood flow and musculovascular events. *J. Urol.* 142 (1989): 56–61.

Karacan, I., R. L. Williams, J. I. Thornby, and P. J. Salis. Sleep-related penile tumescence as a function of age. *Am. J. Psychiatry* 132 (1975): 932–37.

Lavoisier, P., J. Proulx, F. Courtois, and F. de Carufel. Bulbocavernosus reflex: its validity as a diagnostic test of neurogenic impotence. *J. Urol.* 141 (1989): 311–14.

Lehman, T. P., and J. J. Jacobs. Etiology of diabetic impotence. *J. Urol.* 129 (1983): 291–94.

Lipson, L. L. Special problems in treatment of hypertension in the patient with diabetes mellitus. *Arch. Intern. Med.* 144 (1984): 1829–31.

Marshall, P., D. Surridge, and N. Delva. The role of nocturnal penile tumescence in differentiating between organic and psychogenic impotence: the first stage of validation. *Arch. Sex. Behav.* 10 (1981): 1–10.

Phelps, G., M. Brown, J. Chen, et al. Sexual experience and plasma testosterone levels in male veterans after spinal cord injury. *Arch. Phys. Med. Rehabil.* 64 (1983): 47–52.

Reynolds, C. F., III, M. E. Thase, R. Jennings, et al. Nocturnal penile tumescence in healthy 20- to 59-year-olds: a revisit. *Sleep* 12 (1989): 368–72.

Schiavi, R. C., C. Fisher, D. White, P. Beers, and R. Szechter. Pituitary-gonadal function during sleep in men with erectile impotence and normal controls. *Psychosom. Med.* 46 (1984): 239–54.

Siroky, M. B., D. S. Sax, and R. J. Krane. Sacral signal tracing: the electrophysiology of the bulbocavernosus reflex. *J. Urol.* 122 (1979): 661–64.

Thase, M. E., C. F. Reynolds III, J. R. Jennings, et al. Diagnostic performance of nocturnal penile tumescence studies in healthy, dysfunctional (impotent), and depressed men. *Psychiatry Research* 26 (1988): 79–87.

Valleroy, M. L., and G. H. Kraft. Sexual dysfunction in multiple sclerosis. *Arch. Phys. Med. Rehabil.* 65 (1984): 125–28.

Velcek, D. Discogenic impotence. *Int. J. Impotence Res.* 1 (1989): 95–113.

Wasserman, M. D., C. P. Pollak, A. J. Spielman, and E. D. Weitzman. The differential diagnosis of impotence. The measurement of nocturnal penile tumescence. *JAMA* 243 (1980): 2038–42.

Wincze, J. P., S. Bansal, D. Malhotra, A. Balko, J. G. Susset, and M. Malmud. A comparison of nocturnal penile tumescence and penile response to erotic stimulation during waking states in comprehensively diagnosed groups of males experiencing erectile difficulties. *Arch. Sex. Behav.* 17 (1988): 333–48.

Chapter 7. The Flow of Blood: Arteries and Veins

Abelson, D. Diagnostic value of the penile pulse and blood pressure: a Doppler study of impotence in diabetics. *J. Urol.* 113 (1975): 636–39.

Bar-Moshe, O., and M. Vandendris. Treatment of impotence due to perineal venous leakage by ligation of crura penis. *J. Urol.* 139 (1988): 1217–19.

Bond, R. E. Distance bicycling may cause ischemic neuropathy of the penis. *Physician Sportsmed.* 3 (1975): 54–56.

Bookstein, J. J., and A. L. Lurie. Selective penile venography: anatomical and hemodynamic observations. *J. Urol.* 140 (1988): 55–60.

Buvat, J., A. Lemaire, M. Buvat-Herbaut, J. D. Guieu, J. P. Bailleul, and P. Fossati. Comparative investigations in 26 impotent and 26 nonimpotent diabetic patients. *J. Urol.* 133 (1985): 34–38.

Chiu, R. C., D. Lidstone, and P. E. Blundell. Predictive power of penile/brachial index in diagnosing male sexual impotence. *J. Vasc. Surg.* 4 (1986): 251–56.

DePalma, R. G., H. A. Emsellem, C. M. Edwards, et al. A screening sequence for vasculogenic impotence. *J. Vasc. Surg.* 5 (1987): 228–36.

Engel, G., S. J. Burnham, and M. F. Carter. Penile blood pressure in the evaluation of erectile impotence. *Fertil. Steril.* 30 (1978): 687–90.

Goldstein, I., M. B. Siroky, R. L. Nath, T. N. McMillian, J. O. Menzoian, and R. J. Krane. Vasculogenic impotence: role of the pelvic steal test. *J. Urol.* 128 (1982): 300–306.

Karacan, I., P. J. Salis, M. Hirshkowitz, R. E. Borreson, E. Narter, and R. L. Williams. Erectile dysfunction in hypertensive men: sleep-related erections, penile blood flow and musculovascular events. *J. Urol.* 142 (1989): 56–61.

Kedia, K. R. Vasculogenic impotence: diagnosis and objective evaluation using quantitative segmental pulse volume recorder. *Br. J. Urol.* 56 (1984): 516–20.

Kerstein, M. D., S. A. Gould, E. French-Sherry, et al. Perineal trauma and vasculogenic impotence. *J. Urol.* 127 (1982): 57.

Lewis, R. W. Venous surgery for impotence. *Urol. Clin. North Am.* 15 (1988): 115–21.

Michal, V., R. Kramar, and J. Pospichal. External iliac "steal syndrome." *J. Cardiovasc. Surg.* 19 (1978): 355–57.

Shaw, W. W., and A. W. Zorgniotti. Surgical techniques in penile revascularization. *Urology* 23 (1984): 76–78.

Virag, R. Pelvic steal syndrome. An appraisal illustrated by clinical and haemodynamic data on seven cases. *VASA* 10 (1980): 304–7.

Virag, R., P. Bouilly, and D. Frydman. Is impotence an arterial disorder? A study of risk factors in 440 impotent men. *Lancet* 1 (1985): 181–84.

Zorgniotti, A. W., G. Rossi, G. Padula, and R. D. Makovsky. Diagnosis and therapy of vasculogenic impotence. *J. Urol.* 123 (1980): 674–77.

Chapter 8. Hormones Regulate Male Sexual Function

Baskin, H. J. Endocrinologic evaluation of impotence. *South. Med. J.* 82 (1989): 446–49.

Blackwell, R. E., and R. Guillemin. Hypothalamic control of adenohypophyseal secretions. *Ann. Rev. Physiol.* 35 (1973): 357–90.

Blumer, D., and A. E. Walker. Sexual behaviour in temporal lobe epilepsy. *Arch. Neurol.* 16 (1967): 37–43.

Bobrow, N. A., J. Money, and V. G. Lewis. Delayed puberty, eroticism, and sense of smell: a psychological study of hypogonadotropinism, osmatic and anosmatic (Kallmann's syndrome). *Arch. Sex. Behav.* 1 (1971): 329–44.

Carter, J. N., J. E. Tyson, G. Tolis, S. Van Vliet, C. Faiman, and H. G. Friesen. Prolactin-secreting tumors and hypogonadism in 22 men. *N. Engl. J. Med.* 299 (1978): 847–52.

Chopra, I. J., and D. Tulchinsky. Status of estrogen androgen balance in hyperthyroid men with Graves' disease. *J. Clin. Endocrinol. Metab.* 38 (1974): 269–77.

Franks, S., H. S. Jacobs, N. Martin, and J. D. Nabarro. Hyperprolactinaemia and impotence. *Clin. Endocrinol.* 8 (1978): 277–87.

Hierons, R., and M. Saunders. Impotence in patients with temporal-lobe lesions. *Lancet* 2 (1966): 761–64.

Hill, T. C., A. L. Holman, R. Levett, et al. Initial experience with SPECT (single photon computerized tomography) of the brain using N-isopropyl I-123 iodoamphetamine (concise communication). *J. Nucl. Med.* 23 (1982): 191–95.

Johnson, J. Sexual impotence and the limbic system. *Br. J. Psychiat.* 111 (1965): 300–303.

Kidd, G. S., A. R. Glass, and R. A. Vigersky. The hypothalamic-pituitary-testicular axis in thyrotoxicosis. *J. Clin. Endocrinol. Metab.* 48 (1979): 798–802.

Linde, R., G. C. Doelle, N. Alexander, et al. Reversible inhibition of testicular steroidogenesis and spermatogenesis by a potent gonadotropin-releasing hormone agonist in normal men. An approach toward the development of a male contraceptive. *N. Engl. J. Med.* 305 (1981): 663–67.

McBride, R. L., and J. Sutin. Amygdaloid and pontine projections to the ventromedial nucleus of the hypothalamus *Comp. Neur.* 174 (1977): 377–96.

Nagulesparen, M., V. Ang, and J. S. Jenkins. Bromocriptine treatment of males with pituitary tumours, hyperprolactinaemia, and hypogonadism. *Clin. Endocrinol.* 9 (1978): 73–79.

Prescott, R. W. G., P. Kendall-Taylor, K. Hall, et al. Hyperprolactinaemia in men—response to bromocriptine therapy. *Lancet* 1 (1982): 245–49.

Santen, R. J., and C. W. Bardin. Episodic luteinizing hormone secretion in man: pulse analysis, clinical interpretation, physiologic mechanisms. *J. Clin. Invest.* 52 (1973): 2617–28.

Slag, M. F., J. E. Morley, M. K. Elson, et al. Impotence in medical clinic outpatients. *JAMA* 249 (1983): 1736–40.

Spark, R. F. Neuroendocrinology and impotence. *Ann. Int. Med.* 98 (1983): 103–5.

Spark, R. F., R. A. White, and P. B. Connolly. Impotence is not always psychogenic: newer insights into hypothalamic-pituitary-gonadal dysfunction. *JAMA* 243 (1980): 750–55.

Spark, R. F., G. O'Reilly, C. A. Wills, B. J. Ransil, and R. Bergland. Hyperprolactinaemia in males with and without pituitary macroadenomas. *Lancet* 2 (1982): 129–32.

Spark, R. F., C. A. Wills, and H. Royal. Hypogonadism, hyperprolactinaemia, and temporal lobe epilepsy in hyposexual men. *Lancet* 1 (1984): 413–17.

Veldhuis, J. D., A. D. Rogol, M. L. Johnson, and M. L. Dufau. Endogenous opiates modulate the pulsatile secretion of biologically active luteinizing hormone in man. *J. Clin. Invest.* 72 (1983): 2031–40.

Winters, S. J., R. S. Mecklenburg, and R. J. Sherins. Hypothalamic function in men with hypogonadotrophic hypogonadism. *Clin. Endocrinol.* 8 (1978): 417–26.

Wortsman, J., W. Rosner, and M. L. Dufau. Abnormal testicular function in men with primary hypothyroidism. *Am. J. Med.* 82 (1987): 207–12.

Yamada, T., and M. A. Greer. The effect of bilateral ablation of the amygdala on endocrine function in the rat. *Endocrinology* 66 (1960): 565–74.

Chapter 9. Medications, Chemicals, and Potency

Apter, A., Z. Dickerman, N. Gonen, et al. Effect of chlorpromazine on hypothalamic-pituitary-gonadal function in 10 adolescent schizophrenic boys. *Am. J. Psychiatry* 140 (1983): 1586–91.

Bansal, S. Sexual dysfunction in hypertensive men: a critical review of the literature. *Hypertension* 12 (1988): 1–10.

Brenner, J., D. Vugrin, and W. F. Whitmore, Jr. Effect of treatment on fertility and sexual function in males with metastatic non-seminomatous germ cell tumors of testis. *Am. J. Clin. Oncol.* 8 (1985): 178–82.

Carson, C. C., and R. D. Mino. Priapism associated with trazodone therapy. *J. Urol.* 139 (1988): 369–70.

Clonidine (Catapres) and other drugs causing sexual dysfunction. *Med. Lett. Drugs Ther.* 19 (1977): 81–82.

Cocores, J. A., N. S. Miller, A. C. Pottash, and M. S. Gold. Sexual dysfunction in abusers of cocaine and alcohol. *Am. J. Drug Alcohol Abuse* 14 (1988): 169–73.

Colin Jones, D. G., M. J. Langman, D. H. Lawson, and M. P. Vessey. Postmarketing surveillance of the safety of cimetidine: twelve-month morbidity report. *Q. J. Med.* 54 (1985): 253–68.

Condra, M., A. Morales, J. A. Owen, D. H. Surridge, and J. Fenemore. Prevalence and significance of tobacco smoking in impotence. *Urology* 27 (1986): 495–98.

Cooper, A. J. Factors in male sexual inadequacy: a review. *J. Nerv. Ment. Dis.* 149 (1969): 337–59.

Croog, S. H., S. Levine, A. Sudilovsky, R. M. Baume, and J. Clive. Sexual symptoms in hypertensive patients: a clinical trial of antihypertensive medications. *Arch. Intern. Med.* 148 (1988): 788–94.

Croog, S. H., S. Levine, M. A. Testa, et al. The effects of antihypertensive therapy on the quality of life. *N. Engl. J. Med.* 314 (1986): 1657–64.

Dawley, H. H., Jr., D. K. Winstead, A. S. Baxter, and J. R. Gay. An attitude survey of the effects of marijuana on sexual enjoyment. *J. Clin. Psychol.* 35 (1979): 212–17.

Drugs and male sexual function. Editorial, *Br. Med. J.* 2 (1979): 883–84.

Forsberg, L., B. Gustavii, T. Hojerback, and A. M. Olsson. Impotence, smoking, and beta-blocking drugs. *Fertil. Steril.* 31 (1979): 589–91.

Fossa, S. D., S. Ous, T. Abyholm, and M. Loeb. Post-treatment fertility in patients with testicular cancer. I. Influence of retroperitoneal lymph dissection on ejaculatory potency. *Br. J. Urol.* 57 (1985): 204–9.

Gilbert, D. G., R. L. Hagen, and J. A. D'Agostino. The effects of cigarette smoking on human sexual potency. *Addict. Behav.* 11 (1986): 431–34.

Glass, R. M. Ejaculatory impairment from both phenelzine and imipramine, with tinnitus from phenelzine. *J. Clin. Psychopharmacol.* 1 (1981): 152–54.

Goldstein, I., M. I. Feldman, P. J. Deckers, R. K. Babayan, and R. J. Krane. Radiation-associated impotence. A clinical study of its mechanism. *JAMA* 251 (1984): 903–10.

Goldwasser, B., I. Madgar, P. Jonas, B. Lunenfeld, and M. Many. Imipramine for the treatment of sterility in patients following retroperitoneal lymph node dissection. *Andrologia* 15 (1983): 588–91.

Gossop, M. R., R. Stern, and P. H. Connell. Drug dependence and sexual dysfunction: a comparison of intravenous users of narcotics and oral users of amphetamines. *Br. J. Psychiatry* 124 (1974): 431–34.

Gwee, M. C., and L. S. Cheah. Actions of cimetidine and ranitidine at some cholinergic sites: implications in toxicolocy and anesthesia. *Life Sci.* 39 (1986): 383–88.

Harrison, W. M., J. G. Rabkin, A. A. Ehrhardt, et al. Effects of antidepressant medication on sexual function: a controlled study. *J. Clin. Psychopharmacol.* 6 (1986): 144–49.

Herman, J. B., A. W. Brotman, M. H. Pollack, W. E. Falk, J. Biederman, and J. F. Rosenbaum. Fluoxetine-induced sexual dysfunction. *J. Clin. Psychiatry* 51 (1990): 25–27.

Jensen, R. T., M. J. Collen, K. E. McArthur, et al. Comparison of the effectiveness of ranitidine and cimetidine in inhibiting acid secretion in patients with gastric hypersecretory states. *Am. J. Med.* 77 (1984): 90–105.

Jensen, R. T., M. J. Collen, S. J. Pandol, et al. Cimetidine-induced impotence and breast changes in patients with gastric hypersecretory states. *N. Engl. J. Med.* 308 (1983): 883–87.

Juenemann, K. P., T. F. Lue, J. A. Luo, N. L. Benowitz, M. Abozeid, and E. A. Tanagho. The effect of cigarette smoking on penile erection. *J. Urol.* 138 (1987): 438–41.

Kline, M. D. Fluoxetine and anorgasmia. Letter, *Am. J. Psychiatry* 146 (1989): 804–5.

Korenman, S. G. Clinical assessment of drug-induced impairment of sexual function in men. *Chest* 83 (1983): 391–92.

Kowalski, A., R. O. Stanley, L. Dennerstein, G. Burrows, and K. P. Maguire. The sexual side effects of antidepressant medication: a double-blind comparison of two antidepressants in a nonpsychiatric population. *Br. J. Psychiatry* 147 (1985): 413–18.

Lin, S. N., P. C. Yu, M. C. Yang, L. S. Chang, B. N. Chiang, and J. S. Kuo. Local suppressive effect of clonidine on penile erection in the dog. *J. Urol.* 139 (1988): 849–52.

Lipson, L. L. Special problems in treatment of hypertension in the patient with diabetes mellitus. *Arch. Intern. Med.* 144 (1984): 1829–31.

————. Treatment of hypertension in diabetic men: problems with sexual dysfunction. *Am. J. Cardiol.* 53 (1984): 46A–50A.

Melman, A., J. Fersel, and P. Weinstein. Further studies on the effect of chronic alpha-methyldopa administration upon the central nervous system and sexual function in male rats. *J. Urol.* 132 (1984): 804–8.

Mendelson, J. H., N. K. Mello, S. K. Teoh, J. Ellingboe, and J. Cochin. Cocaine effects on pusatile secretion of anterior pituitary, gonadal, and adrenal hormones. *J. Clin. Endocrinol. Metab.* 69 (1989): 1256–60.

Mitchell, J. E., and M. K. Popkin. Antidepressant drug therapy and sexual dysfunction in men: a review. *J. Clin. Psychopharmacol.* 3 (1983): 76–79.

————. Antipsychotic drug therapy and sexual dysfunction in men. *Am. J. Psychiatry* 139 (1982): 633–37.

Moss, H. B., and W. R. Procci. Sexual dysfunction associated with oral antihypertensive medication: a critical survey of the literature. *Gen. Hosp. Psychiatry* 4 (1982): 121–29.

Newman, H. F., and H. Marcus. Erectile dysfunction in diabetes and hypertension. *Urology* 26 (1985): 135–37.

Nijman, J. M., S. Jager, P. W. Boer, J. Kremer, J. Oldhoff, and H. S. Koops. The treatment of ejaculation disorders after retroperitoneal lymph node dissection. *Cancer* 50 (1982): 2967–71.

Peden, N. R., J. M. Cargill, M. C. Browning, J. H. Saunders, and K. G. Wormsley. Male sexual dysfunction during treatment with cimetidine. *Br. Med. J.* 1 (1979): 659.

Quirk, K. C., and T. R. Einarson. Sexual dysfunction and clomipramine. *Can. J. Psychiatry* 27 (1982): 228–31.

Rabkin, J. G., F. M. Quitkin, P. McGrath, W. Harrison, and E. Tricamo. Adverse reactions to monoamine oxidase inhibitors. Part II. Treatment correlates and clinical management. *J. Clin. Psychopharmacol.* 5 (1985): 2–9.

Report of Medical Research Council Working Party on Mild to Moderate Hypertension. Adverse reactions to bendrofluazide and propranolol for the treatment of mild hypertension. *Lancet* 2 (1981): 539–43.

Reynolds, C. F., III, E. Frank, M. E. Thase, et al. Assessment of sexual function in depressed, impotent, and healthy men: factor analysis of a brief sexual function questionnaire for men. *Psychiatry Res.* 24 (1988): 231–50.

Scharf, M. B., and D. W. Mayleben. Comparative effects of prazosin and hydrochlorothiazide on sexual function in hypertensive men. *Am. J. Med.* 86 (1989): 110–12.

Schneider, J., and H. Kaffarnik. Impotence in patients treated with clofibrate. *Atherosclerosis* 21 (1975): 455–57.

Segraves, R. T. Effects of psychotropic drugs on human erection and ejaculation. *Arch. Gen. Psychiatry* 46 (1989): 275–84.

Segraves, R. T., R. Madsen, C. S. Carter, and J. M. Davis. Erectile dysfunction associated with pharmacological agents. In R. T. Segraves and H. W. Schoenberg, eds. *Diagnosis and treatment of erectile disturbances: a guide for clinicians.* New York: Plenum, 1985.

Sjogren, K., and A. R. Fugl-Meyer. Some factors influencing quality of sexual life after myocardial infarction. *Int. Rehabil. Med.* 5 (1983): 197–201.

Smith, D. E., D. R. Wesson, and M. Apter-Marsh. Cocaine- and alcohol-induced sexual dysfunction in patients with addictive disease. *J. Psychoactive Drugs* 16 (1984): 359–61.

Thase, M. E., C. F. Reynolds III, J. R. Jennings, et al. Nocturnal penile tumescence is diminished in depressed men. *Biol. Psychiatry* 24 (1988): 33–46.

Van Thiel, D. H., J. S. Gavaler, P. K. Eagon, Y. B. Chiao, C. F. Cobb, and R. Lester. Alcohol and sexual function. *Pharmacol. Biochem. Behav.* 13 (1980): 125–29.

Wein, A. J., and K. N. Van Arsdalen. Drug-induced male sexual dysfunction. *Urol. Clin. North Am.* 15 (1988): 23–31.

Chapter 10. Prostate Surgery and Other Medical Problems

Bolt, J. W., C. Evans, and V. R. Marshall. Sexual dysfunction after prostatectomy. *Br. J. Urol.* 59 (1987): 319–22.

Finkle, A. L., and D. V. Prian. Sexual potency in elderly men before and after prostatectomy. *JAMA* 196 (1966): 139–43.

Finkle, A. L., and S. P. Taylor. Sexual potency after radical prostatectomy. *J. Urol.* 125 (1981): 350–52.

Levison, V. The effect on fertility, libido and sexual function of postoperative radiotherapy and chemotherapy for cancer of the testicle. *Clin. Radiol.* 37 (1986): 161–64.

Moller-Nielsen, C., E. Lundhus, B. Moller-Madsen, et al. Sexual life following "minimal" and "total" transurethral prostatic resection. *Urol. Int.* 40 (1985): 3–4.

Walsh, P. C. Radical prostatectomy, preservation of sexual function, cancer control. The controversy. *Urol. Clin. North Am.* 14 (1987): 663–73.

Walsh, P. C., J. I. Epstein, and F. C. Lowe. Potency following radical prostatectomy with wide unilateral excision of the neurovascular bundle. *J. Urol.* 138 (1987): 823–27.

Wasserman, M. D., C. P. Pollak, A. J. Spielman, and E. D. Weitzman. Impaired nocturnal erections and impotence following transurethral prostatectomy. *Urology* 15 (1980): 552–55.

Weldon, V. E., and F. R. Tavel. Potency-sparing radical perineal prostatectomy: anatomy, surgical technique and initial results. *J. Urol.* 140 (1988): 559–62.

Chapter 11. Psychologic Factors Affecting Potency and Ejaculation

Beck, J. G., and D. H. Barlow. The effects of anxiety and attentional focus on sexual responding—II. Cognitive and affective patterns in erectile dysfunction. *Behav. Res. Ther.* 24 (1986): 19–26.

Chesney, A. P., P. E. Blakeney, C. M. Cole, and R. A. Chan. A comparison of couples who have sought sex therapy with couples who have not. *J. Sex. Marital Ther.* 7 (1981): 131–40.

Daniel, D. G., V. Abernethy, and W. R. Oliver. Correlations between female sex roles and attitudes toward male sexual dysfunction in thirty women. *J. Sex. Marit. Ther.* 10 (1984): 160–69.

Dekker, J., W. Everaerd, and N. Verhelst. Attending to stimuli or to images of sexual feelings: effects on sexual arousal. *Behav. Res. Ther.* 23 (1985): 139–49.

Derogatis, L. R., J. K. Meyer, and S. Kourlesis. Psychiatric diagnosis and psychological symptoms in impotence. *Hillside Journal of Clinical Psychiatry* 7 (1985): 120–33.

Farkas, G. M., L. F. Sine, and I. M. Evans. Personality, sexuality, and demographc differences between volunteers and nonvolunteers for a laboratory study of male sexual behavior. *Arch. Sex. Behav.* 7 (1978): 513–20.

Hall, K. S., Y. Binik, and E. Di Tomasso. Concordance between physiological and subjective measures of sexual arousal. *Behav. Res. Ther.* 23 (1985): 297–303.

Kaplan, H. S. *The new sex therapy: active treatment of dysfunctions.* New York: Brunner/Mazel, 1974.

Kinsey, A. C., W. B. Pomeroy, and C. E. Martin. *Sexual behavior in the human male.* Philadelphia: Saunders, 1948.

Kockott, G., W. Feil, D. Revenstorf, J. Aldenhoff, and U. Besinger. Symptomatology and psychological aspects of male sexual inadequacy: results of an experimental study. *Archives of Sexual Behavior* 9 (1980): 457–75.

Levine, S. B. The psychological evaluation and therapy of psychogenic impotence. In R. T. Segraves and H. W. Schoenberg, eds. *Diagnosis and treatment of erectile disturbances: a guide for clinicians.* New York: Plenum, 1985.

Masters, W., and V. Johnson. *Human Sexual Inadequacy.* Boston: Little, Brown, 1970.

————. *Human Sexual Response.* Boston: Little, Brown, 1966.

Morse, W. I., and J. M. Morse. Erectile impotence precipitated by organic factors and perpetuated by performance anxiety. *CMA Journal* 127 (1982): 599–601.

Notzer, N., D. Levran, S. Mashiach, and S. Soffer. Effect of religiosity on sex attitudes, experience and contraception among university students. *J. Sex. Marital Ther.* 10 (1984): 57–62.

Reynolds, C. F., III, E. Frank, M. E. Thase, et al. Assessment of sexual function in depressed, impotent, and healthy men: factor analysis of a brief sexual function questionnaire for men. *Psychiatry Res.* 24 (1988): 231–50.

Roose, S. P., A. H. Glassman, B. T. Walsh, and K. Cullen. Reversible loss of nocturnal penile tumescence during depression: a preliminary report. *Neuropsychobiology* 8 (1982): 284–88.

Sakheim, D. K., D. H. Barlow, J. G. Beck, and D. J. Abrahamson. The effect of an increased awareness of erectile cues on sexual arousal. *Behav. Res. Ther.* 22 (1984): 151–58.

Schover, L. R., J. M. Friedman, S. J. Weiler, J. R. Heiman, and J. LoPiccolo. Multiaxial problem-oriented system for sexual dysfunctions. An alternative to DSM-III. *Arch. Gen. Psychiatry* 39 (1982): 614–19.

Segraves, R. T., H. W. Schoenberg, C. K. Zarins, P. Camic, and J. Knopf. Characteristics of erectile dysfunction as a function of medical care system entry point. *Psychosomatic Medicine* 43 (1981): 227–34.

Stief, C. G., W. Bahren, W. Scherb, and H. Gall. Primary erectile dysfunction. *J. Urol.* 141 (1989): 315–19.

Takanami, M., M. Matsuhashi, A. Maki, et al. Evaluation of therapeutic efficacy in psychogenic impotence by means of logarithmic scoring. *Urology* 27 (1986): 309–17.

Weintraub, W., and H. Aronson. Patients in psychoanalysis: some findings related to sex and religion. *Am. J. Orthopsychiatry* 44 (1974): 102–8.

Chapter 12. Penile Implants

Apte, S. M., J. G. Gregory, and M. H. Purcell. The inflatable penile prosthesis, reoperation and patient satisfaction: a comparison of statistics obtained from patient record review with statistics obtained from intensive follow-up search. *J. Urol.* 131 (1984): 894–95.

Barry, J. M. Clinical experience with hinged silicone penile implants for impotence. *J. Urol.* 123 (1980): 178–79.

Benson, R. C., Jr., D. M. Barrett, and D. E. Patterson. The Jonas prosthesis—technical considerations and results. *J. Urol.* 130 (1983): 920–22.

Bertram, R. A., C. C. Carson, and L. F. Altaffer. Severe penile curvature after implantation of an inflatable penile prosthesis. *J. Urol.* 139 (1988): 743–45.

Beutler, L. E., F. B. Scott, R. R. Rogers, Jr., I. Karacan, P. E. Baer, and J. A. Gaines. Inflatable and noninflatable penile prostheses: comparative follow-up evaluation. *Urology* 27 (1986): 136–43.

Brooks, M. B. Forty-two months of experience with the Mentor inflatable penile prosthesis. *J. Urol.* 139 (1988): 48–49.

Carson, C. C., and C. N. Robertson. Late hematogenous infection of penile prostheses. *J. Urol.* 139 (1988): 50–52.

Collins, K. P., and R. H. Hackler. Complications of penile prostheses in the spinal cord injury population. *J. Urol.* 140 (1988): 984–85.

Fallon, B., S. Rosenberg, and D. A. Culp. Long-term followup in patients with an inflatable penile prosthesis. *J. Urol.* 132 (1984): 270–71.

Finney, R. P., J. R. Sharpe, and R. W. Sadlowski. Finney hinged penile implant: experience with 100 cases. *J. Urol.* 124 (1980): 205–7.

Furlow, W. L., and B. Goldwasser. Salvage of the eroded inflatable penile prosthesis: a new concept. *J. Urol.* 138 (1987): 312–14.

Furlow, W. L., B. Goldwasser, and J. C. Gundian. Implantation of model AMS 700 penile prosthesis: long-term results. *J. Urol.* 139 (1988): 741–42.

Furlow, W. L., and R. C. Motley. The inflatable penile prosthesis: clinical experience with a new controlled expansion cyclinder. *J. Urol.* 139 (1988): 945–46.

Gerstenberger, D. L., D. Osborne, and W. L. Furlow. Inflatable penile prosthesis: follow-up study of patient-partner satisfaction. *Urology* 14 (1979): 583–87.

Gregory, J. G., and M. H. Purcell. Scott's inflatable penile prosthesis: evaluation of mechanical survival in the series 700 model. *J. Urol.* 137 (1987): 676–77.

Hollander, J. B., and A. C. Diokno. Success with penile prosthesis from patient's viewpoint. *Urology* 23 (1984): 141–43.

Joseph, D. B., R. C. Bruskewitz, and R. C. Benson, Jr. Long-term evaluation of the inflatable penile prosthesis. *J. Urol.* 131 (1984): 670–73.

Kabalin, J. N., and R. Kessler. Experience with the hydroflex penile prosthesis. *J. Urol.* 141 (1989): 58–59.

――――. Infectious complications of penile prosthesis surgery. *J. Urol.* 139 (1988): 953–55.

Kaufman, J. J. Penile prosthetic surgery under local anesthesia. *J. Urol.* 128 (1982): 1190–91.

Kramarsky-Binkhorst, S. Female partner perception of Small-Carrion implant. *Urology* 12 (1978): 545–48.

Krauss, D. J., D. Bogin, and A. Culebras. The failed penile prosthetic implantation despite technical success. *J. Urol.* 129 (1983): 969–71.

Malloy, T. R., A. J. Wein, and V. L. Carpiniello. Comparison of the inflatable penile and the Small-Carrion prostheses in the surgical treatment of erectile impotence. *J. Urol.* 123 (1980): 678–79.

Montague, D. K. Experience with semirigid rod and inflatable penile prostheses. *J. Urol.* 129 (1983): 967–68.

Pedersen, B., L. Tiefer, M. Ruiz, and A. Melman. Evaluation of patients and partners 1 to 4 years after penile prosthesis surgery. *J. Urol.* 139 (1988): 956–58.

Rossier, A. B., and B. A. Fam. Indication and results of semirigid penile prostheses in spinal cord injury patients: long-term followup. *J. Urol.* 131 (1984): 59–62.

Schlamowitz, K. E., L. E. Beutler, F. B. Scott, I. Karacan, and C. Ware. Reactions to the implantation of an inflatable penile prosthesis among psychogenically and organically impotent men. *J. Urol.* 129 (1983): 295–98.

Schover, L. R., and A. C. von Eschenbach. Sex therapy and the penile prosthesis: a synthesis. *J. Sex. Marital Ther.* 11 (1985): 57–66.

Scott, F. B., I. J. Fishman, and J. K. Light. A decade of experience with the inflatable penile prosthesis. *World J. Urol.* 1 (1983): 244–50.

Stanisic, T. H., J. C. Dean, J. M. Donovan, and L. E. Beutler. Clinical experience with a self-contained inflatable penile implant: the flexi-flate. *J. Urol.* 139 (1988): 947–50.

Steege, J. F., A. L. Stout, and C. C. Carson. Patient satisfaction in Scott and Small-Carrion penile implant recipients: a study of 52 patients. *Archives of Sexual Behavior* 15 (1986): 393–99.

Stewart, T. D. Penile prosthesis: potential value of medical psychiatric assessment and psychotherapy. *Psychother. Psychosom.* 44 (1985): 18–24.

Thomalla, J. V., S. T. Thompson, R. G. Rowland, and J. J. Mulcahy. Infectious complications of penile prosthetic implants. *J. Urol.* 138 (1987): 65–67.

Wilson, S. K., G. E. Wahman, and J. L. Lange. Eleven years of experience with the inflatable penile prosthesis. *J. Urol.* 139 (1988): 951–52.

Chapter 13. Penile Injection

Althof, S. E., L. A. Turner, S. B. Levine, et al. Intracavernosal injection in the treatment of impotence: a prospective study of sexual, psychological, and marital functioning. *J. Sex. Marital Ther.* 13 (1987): 155–67.

Bahnson, R. R., and W. J. Catalona. Papaverine testing of impotent patients following nerve-sparing radical prostatectomy. *J. Urol.* 139 (1988): 773–74.

Brindley, G. S. Cavernosal alpha-blockade: a new technique for investigating and treating erectile impotence. *Brit. J. Psychiat.* 143 (1983): 332–37.

Buvat, J., M. Buvat-Herbaut, J. L. Dehaene, and A. Lemaire. Is intracavernous injection of papaverine a reliable screening test for vascular impotence? *J. Urol.* 135 (1986): 476–78.

Corriere, J. N., Jr., I. J. Fishman, G. S. Benson, and C. E. Carlton, Jr. Development of fibrotic penile lesions secondary to the intracorporeal injection of vasoactive agents. *J. Urol.* 140 (1988): 615–17.

Girdley, F. M., R. C. Bruskewitz, J. Feyzi, P. H. Graversen, and T. C. Gasser. Intracavernous self-injection for impotence: a long-term therapeutic option? Experience in 78 patients. *J. Urol.* 140 (1988): 972–74.

Glina, S., A. C. Reichelt, P. P. Leao, and J. M. Dos Reis. Impact of cigarette smoking on papaverine-induced erection. *J. Urol.* 140 (1988): 523–24.

Hu, K. N., C. Burks, and W. C. Christy. Fibrosis of tunica albuginea: complication of long-term intracavernous pharmacological self-injection. *J. Urol.* 138 (1987): 404–5.

Ishii, N., H. Watanabe, C. Irisawa, et al. Intracavernous injection of prostaglandin E_1 for the treatment of erectile impotence. *J. Urol.* 141 (1989): 323–25.

Juenemann, K. P., and P. Alken. Pharmacotherapy of erectile dysfunction: a review. *Int. J. Impotence Res.* 1 (1989): 71–93.

Levine, S. B., S. E. Althof, L. A. Turner, et al. Side effects of self-administration of intracavernous papaverine and phentolamine for the treatment of impotence. *J. Urol.* 141 (1989): 54–57.

Sidi, A. A. Vasoactive intracavernous pharmacotherapy. *Urol. Clin. North Am.* 15 (1988): 95–101.

Sidi, A. A., J. S. Cameron, L. M. Duffy, and P. H. Lange. Intra-cavernous drug-induced erections in the management of male erectile dysfunction: experience with 100 patients. *J. Urol.* 135 (1986): 704–6.

Sidi, A. A., J. S. Cameron, D. D. Dykstra, Y. Reinberg, and P. H. Lange. Vasoactive intracavernous pharmacotherapy for the treat-ment of erectile impotence in men with spinal cord injury. *J. Urol.* 138 (1987): 539–42.

Stackl, W., R. Hasun, and M. Marberger. Intracavernous injec-tion of prostaglandin E₁ in impotent men. *J. Urol.* 140 (1988): 66–68.

Tullii, R. E., M. Degni, and A. F. C. Pinto. Fibrosis of the cavern-ous bodies following intracavernous auto-injection of vasoactive drugs. *Int. J. Impotence Res.* 1 (1989): 49–54.

Virag, R. About pharmacologically induced prolonged erection. *Lancet* 1 (1985): 519–20.

Wespes, E., C. Delcour, C. Rondeux, J. Struyven, and C. C. Schul-man. The erectile angle: objective criterion to evaluate the pa-paverine test in impotence. *J. Urol.* 138 (1987): 1171–73.

Winter, C. C., and G. McDowell. Experience with 105 patients with priapism: update review of all aspects. *J. Urol.* 140 (1988): 980–83.

Zorgniotti, A. W., and R. S. Lefleur. Auto-injection of the corpus cavernosum with a vasoactive drug combination for vasculogenic impotence. *J. Urol.* 133 (1985): 39–41.

Chapter 14. Other Therapies

Abbasi, A. A., A. S. Prasad, J. Ortega, E. Congco, and D. Oberleas. Gonadal function abnormalities in sickle cell anemia. Studies in adult male patients. *Ann. Int. Med.* 85 (1976): 601–5.

Abbasi, A. A., A. S. Prasad, P. Rabbani, and E. DuMouchelle. Ex-perimental zinc deficiency in man. Effect on testicular function. *J. Lab. Clin. Med.* 96 (1980): 544–50.

Hartoma, T. R., K. Nahoul, and A. Netter. Zinc, plasma androgens and male sterility. *Lancet* 2 (1977): 1125–26.

Mahajan, S. K., A. S. Prasad, P. Rabbani, W. A. Briggs, and F. D. McDonald. Zinc deficiency: a reversible complication of uremia. *Am. J. Clin. Nutr.* 36 (1982): 1177–83.

Marder, H. K., L. S. Srivastava, and S. Burstein. Hypergonado-tropism in peripubertal boys with chronic renal failure. *Pediatrics* 72 (1983): 384–89.

Margolis, R., P. Prieto, L. Stein, and S. Chinn. Statistical summary of 10,000 male cases using Afrodex in treatment of impotence. *Curr. Ther. Res.* 13 (1971): 616–22.

Marmar, J. L., T. J. DeBenedictis, and D. E. Praiss. The use of a vacuum constrictor device to augment a partial erection following an intracavernous injection. *J. Urol.* 140 (1988): 975–79.

Morales, A., D. H. C. Surridge, P. G. Marshall, and J. Fenemore. Nonhormonal pharmacological treatment of organic impotence. *J. Urol.* 128 (1982): 45–47.

Nadig, P. W. Six years' experience with the vacuum constriction device. *Int. J. Impotence Res.* 1 (1989): 55–58.

Nadig, P. W., J. C. Ware, and R. Blumoff. Noninvasive device to produce and maintain an erection-like state. *Urology* 27 (1986): 126–31.

Witherington, R. Vacuum constriction device for management of erectile impotence. *J. Urol.* 141 (1989): 320–22.

Yohimbine: time for resurrection? Editorial, *Lancet* 2 (1986): 1194–95.

Chapter 15. Male Fertility and Infertility

Spark, R. F. *The infertile male—the clinician's guide to diagnosis and treatment.* New York: Plenum, 1988.

Chapter 16. Is There a Male Climacteric?

Bremner, W. J., M. V. Vitiello, and P. N. Prinz. Loss of circadian rhythmicity in blood testosterone levels with aging in normal men. *J. Clin. Endocrinol. Metab.* 56 (1983): 1278–81.

Davidson, J. M., J. J. Chen, L. Crapo, G. D. Gray, W. J. Greenleaf, and J. A. Catania. Hormonal changes and sexual function in aging men. *J. Clin. Endocrinol. Metab.* 57 (1983): 71–77.

Deslypere, J. P., J. M. Kaufman, T. Vermeulen, D. Vogelaers, J. L. Vandalem, and A. Vermeulen. Influence of age on pulsatile luteinizing hormone release and responsiveness of the gonadotrophs to sex hormone feedback in men. *J. Clin. Endocrinol. Metab.* 64 (1987): 68–73.

Deslypere, J. P., and A. Vermeulen. Leydig cell function in normal men: effect of age, life-style, residence, diet, and activity. *J. Clin. Endocrinol. Metab.* 59 (1984): 955–62.

Hallberg, M. C., R. G. Wieland, E. M. Zorn, B. H. Furst, and J. M. Wieland. Impaired Leydig cell reserve and altered serum androgen binding in the aging male. *Fertil. Steril.* 27 (1976): 812–14.

Harman, S. M., and P. D. Tsitouras. Reproductive hormones in aging men. I. Measurement of sex steroids, basal luteinizing hormone, and Leydig cell response to human chorionic gonadotropin. *J. Clin. Endocrinol. Metab.* 51 (1980): 35–40.

Harman, S. M., P. D. Tsitouras, P. T. Costa, and M. R. Blackman. Reproductive hormones in aging men. II. Basal pituitary gonadotropins and gonadotropin responses to luteinizing hormone-releasing hormone. *J. Clin. Endocrinol. Metab.* 54 (1982): 547–51.

Heller, C. G., and G. B. Myers. The male climacteric, its symptomatology, diagnosis and treatment. *JAMA* 126 (1944): 472–77.

Kaplan, H. S. The concept of presbyrectia. *Int. J. Impotence Res.* 1 (1989): 59–65.

Karacan, I., R. L. Williams, J. I. Thornby, and P. J. Salis. Sleep-related penile tumescence as a function of age. *Am. J. Psychiatry* 132 (1975): 932–37.

Mulligan, T., S. M. Retchin, V. M. Chinchilli, and C. B. Bettinger. The role of aging and chronic disease in sexual dysfunction. *J. Am. Geriatr. Soc.* 36 (1988): 520–24.

Neaves, W. B., L. Johnson, J. C. Porter, C. R. Parker, Jr., and C. S. Petty. Leydig cell numbers, daily sperm production, and serum gonadotropin levels in aging men. *J. Clin. Endocrinol. Metab.* 59 (1984): 756–63.

Nieschlag, E., U. Lammers, C. W. Freischem, K. Langer, and E. J. Wickings. Reproductive functions in young fathers and grandfathers. *J. Clin. Endocrinol. Metab.* 55 (1982): 676–81.

Tenover, J. S., A. M. Matsumoto, S. R. Plymate, and W. J. Bremner. The effects of aging in normal men on bioavailable testosterone and luteinizing hormone secretion: response to clomiphene citrate. *J. Clin. Endocrinol. Metab.* 65 (1987): 1118–26.

Tsitouras, P. D., C. E. Martin, and S. M. Harman. Relationship of serum testosterone to sexual activity in healthy elderly men. *J. Gerontol.* 37 (1982): 288–93.

Urban, R. J., J. D. Veldhuis, R. M. Blizzard, and M. L. Dufau. Attenuated release of biologically active luteinizing hormone in healthy aging men. *J. Clin. Invest.* 81 (1988): 1020–29.

Vermeulen, A., J. P. Deslypere, and J. M. Kaufman. Influence of antiopioids on luteinizing hormone pulsatility in aging men. *J. Clin. Endocrinol. Metab.* 68 (1989): 68–72.

Vermeulen, A., R. Rubens, and L. Verdonck. Testosterone secretion and metabolism in male senescence. *J. Clin. Endocrinol. Metab.* 34 (1972): 730–35.

Warner, B. A., M. L. Dufau, and R. J. Santen. Effects of aging and illness on the pituitary testicular axis in men: qualitative as well as quantitative changes in luteinizing hormone. *J. Clin. Endocrinol. Metab.* 60 (1985): 263–68.

Werner, A. A. The male climacteric. *JAMA* 112 (1939): 1441–43.

Winters, S. J., R. J. Sherins, and P. Troen. The gonadotropin-suppressive activity of androgen is increased in elderly men. *Metabolism* 33 (1984): 1052–59.

Zumoff, B., G. W. Strain, J. Kream, et al. Age variation of the 24-hour mean plasma concentrations of androgens, estrogens, and gonadotropins in normal adult men. *J. Clin. Endocrinol. Metab.* 54 (1982): 534–38.

Index